Preparing a health care workforce for the 21st century

THE CHALLENGE OF CHRONIC CONDITIONS

World Health Organization
Noncommunicable Diseases and Mental Health Cluster
Chronic Diseases and Health Promotion Department

WHO Library Cataloguing-in-Publication Data

Preparing a health care workforce for the 21st century: the challenge of chronic conditions.

1. Health personnel – education 2. Health personnel – trends 2. Professional competence – standards 3. Competency-based education – organization and administration 4. Patient care 5. Chronic disease I.World Health Organization.

ISBN 92 4 156280 3 (NLM classification: W 18)

Printed in France

Design by Inís: www.inis.ie

P. Schäfer

petra.schaefer@unibas.ch

Table of contents

Acknowledgements

This publication was produced under the overall supervision of Judith Canny (Technical Officer, Health Care for Chronic Conditions, Chronic Diseases and Health Promotion) and JoAnne Epping-Jordan (Coordinator, Health Care for Chronic Conditions, Chronic Diseases and Health Promotion). The principal author was Sheri D. Pruitt (Kaiser Permanente, USA). Rafael Bengoa (Director, Health System Policies and Operations) and Robert Beaglehole (Director, Chronic Diseases and Health Promotion) provided leadership and guidance at different stages of the publication's development.

Case examples were contributed by: Alberto Barcelo, Judith Canny, Joan Dzenowagis, JoAnne Epping-Jordan, Fu Dongbo, Berhane Gebru, Tesfamicael Ghebrehiwet, Wendy Hoy, Holly Ladd, Rashad Massoud, Satu Siiskonen, and the European Respiratory Society Task Force on Integrated Care.

Valuable technical input was received from a range of WHO staff at Headquarters and Regional Offices. In addition, WHO is exceedingly grateful to the many policy-makers, health care leaders, and other experts who gave their time to provide comments and suggestions on this publication at different stages. In particular, WHO would like to acknowledge the valuable input of the World Health Professions Alliance (The World Medical Association, The International Council of Nurses and The International Pharmaceutical Federation), the European Respiratory Society and the International Alliance of Patients' Organizations.

Administrative support for the production of this publication was provided by Elmira Adenova (Health Care for Chronic Conditions, Chronic Diseases and Health Promotion). Photographs were identified and chosen by Elmira Adenova and Aku Kwamie (Health Care for Chronic Conditions, Chronic Diseases and Health Promotion). Editing, graphic design and layout were completed by Inís (www.inis.ie).

The production of this publication was made possible through the generous financial support of the European Respiratory Society.

List of all acronyms and abbreviations used in this report

CDSMP	Chronic Disease Self-Management Programme
COPD	chronic obstructive pulmonary disease
DEHKO	Development Programme for the Prevention and Care of Diabetes
DPP	Diabetes Programme for Pharmacies
ERS	European Respiratory Society
FIP	International Pharmaceutical Federation
HIV/AIDS	human immunodeficiency virus/acquired immune deficiency syndrome
IAPO	International Alliance of Patients' Organizations
ICCC	Innovative Care for Chronic Conditions
ICCP	Integrated Care Programme for Chronic Patients
ICN	International Council of Nurses
ICT	information and communications technology
IMAI	Integrated Management of Adolescent and Adult Illness
PAHO	Pan American Health Organization
PAL	Practical Approach to Lung Health programme
WHO	World Health Organization
WHPA	World Health Professions Alliance
WMA	World Medical Association

Supporting statement: World Medical Association

It is a privilege for the World Medical Association (WMA), the global representative body for physicians, to speak in support of this important World Health Organization (WHO) project. With almost nine million physicians worldwide forming an integral part of the health care workforce, the expansion of the core competencies mentioned in this report will help the medical profession and all other health professionals to provide care for patients suffering from chronic conditions more effectively.

The WMA Declaration of Geneva[1] asserts one of the fundamental principles of medical practice: "The health of my patient will be my first consideration." It is therefore particularly encouraging to see WHO emphasizing the need to make patient-centred care a priority in the development of the health workforce of the 21st century. This will hopefully enable patients suffering from chronic conditions to become active participants, rather than passive recipients, in all aspects of the health care system they are exposed to. This should include the way we develop health care facilities, diagnostic and therapeutic methods, and most important of all, the way in which health professionals partner with their patients to co-manage their chronic health problems on a day-to-day basis.

Another highlight of this report is its focus on partnerships. For too long the care of patients with chronic conditions has taken place in a compartmentalized fashion, often with significant differences in the care plans of hospital, clinic and different health professionals for the same patient. Only effective partnering can overcome this obstacle and improve health results, especially in the prevention of disease. The sophistication of communication technology will certainly enable better partnering and improvement in the quality of care. However, this should not be applied in a manner that would endanger the confidentiality of personal health information, which WMA regards as a fundamental ethical right of the patient.

The section on the measurement of care delivery and outcomes deserves credit. This is a global trend that has especially influenced medical practice

[1] *Declaration of Geneva.* Geneva, World Medical Association, 1948 (http://www.wma.net/e/policy/c8.htm, accessed 22 October 2004).

all over the world, and is to be commended. If a health care delivery system cannot be measured, it cannot be managed, and almost invariably this leads to unnecessary costs and suboptimal care of the individual patients involved. It is constructive and helpful for this WHO project to state that the evidence base for health care delivery is not only derived from randomized clinical trials, but also from what we learn from quality improvement efforts. The best practice examples included in the report further enable health professionals to emulate this in their respective domains.

It is exactly this last point that WMA sees as one of the greatest opportunities of this project. Whereas WHO has ministries of health worldwide as its principal members, the lessons learnt in this project shall be applied mostly in the public health care sectors of the countries represented in WHO. Because health professionals work both in the public and private sectors, they can play a pivotal role in translating the evidence-based improvements resulting from this project into practice. Imagine the synergies and increased effectiveness that can result from such cross-sectoral and interdisciplinary collaboration!

WHO should be encouraged and congratulated on this project. It will be an honour for WMA to participate as partner in helping to care for the patients we jointly serve.

Delon Human
Secretary-General
World Medical Association

Supporting statement: International Council of Nurses

The International Council of Nurses (ICN) strongly endorses this publication and calls on educational and academic institutions, professional organizations such as national nurses' associations, and other stakeholders to use the competencies in training health care providers to meet the care needs of growing populations with chronic conditions.

ICN, as a federation of national nurses' associations in 125 countries, and as the international voice of nurses and nursing, is pleased to see a publication that aims to transform health care workforce training to meet the needs of patients with chronic conditions. ICN particularly welcomes the participatory process in developing this publication.

This document also sets the stage by calling for a new type of partnerships between lay health workers, nurses, pharmacists, dentists, physicians, and allied health professionals. In addition, the publication makes the case for a paradigm shift from the acute care model to a chronic care model, dictated by the current predominance of chronic conditions, including diabetes, heart disease, asthma, cancer, human immunodeficiency virus/acquired immune deficiency syndrome (HIV/AIDS), depression, and physical disabilities. Its central focus on patient-centred care, and the identification of the five core competencies needed to achieve this, is in line with ICN core competencies of both the generalist nurse and the family nurse.[2]

ICN has long been concerned that traditional training in health care focuses largely on the biomedical model of diagnosis and the treatment of acute problems, and neglects the care of the growing population of patients with chronic conditions. Over recent years, ICN has advocated widely for refocusing nursing education programmes towards a continuum of care, encompassing health promotion, disease prevention, acute and chronic care, as well as palliative and rehabilitative care. Thus, the current document is timely and highly pertinent to the health care workforce.

---

[2] *ICN framework and core competencies for the family nurse.* Geneva, International Council of Nurses, 2003.

Among the strongest points of the publication is the identification of a new, expanded training model, based on a set of core competencies that would prepare the health care workforce to care for patients with chronic conditions. The competencies can serve as a starting point for the reform of health training institutions and of centres of higher education.

Judith Oulton
Chief Executive Officer
International Council of Nurses

Supporting statement: International Pharmaceutical Federation

The International Pharmaceutical Federation (FIP) fully supports the basic competencies presented in this document and looks forward to continue working together with WHO, other health professionals and their patients, for better care for patients with chronic conditions, and for the prevention of such conditions.

Pharmacists are health professionals whose role is to help people maintain good health and prevent disease while guaranteeing access to medicines and their best use.

Therapy with prescribed medicines is understood as a collaborative process involving the patient, the physician, the pharmacist and other health care providers. Medicines are primarily self-administered, their success depending therefore upon the active participation of patients. Objective information and guidance is required from health professionals in order to obtain maximum therapeutic benefit and to avoid unwanted side-effects from courses of treatment.

Pharmacists have, consequently, adopted a patient-centred approach in the professional services they provide. This ensures that both patient care and economic aspects are considered and correctly balanced in the interests of the patient, creating an adequate setting for the provision of pharmaceutical care.

The goal of pharmaceutical care is to optimize the patient's health-related quality of life and to achieve positive clinical outcomes. Pharmacists, through the practice of pharmaceutical care, can prevent or stop drug interactions, monitor and prevent, or minimize, adverse drug reactions, and monitor the cost and effectiveness of drug therapy, as well as provide lifestyle counselling to optimize the therapeutic effects of a medication regime. The concept of pharmaceutical care is particularly relevant to special groups, such as the elderly and chronically ill patients.

FIP has drafted a code of ethics[3] to reaffirm and state publicly the principles forming the basis of the roles and responsibilities of pharmacists. These

[3] *FIP statement of professional standards: Code of ethics for pharmacists.* Vancouver, Council of the International Pharmaceutical Federation (FIP), 1997 (http://www.fip.org/pdf/2004codeofethics.pdf, accessed 22 October 2004).

principles, based on moral obligations and values, were established to enable national pharmaceutical organizations to guide pharmacists in their relationships with patients, other health professionals, and society in general.

All practicing pharmacists are obliged to ensure that the service they provide to every patient is of appropriate quality. In 1993, FIP compiled international guidelines for good pharmacy practice[4], with the goal of concretely raising the quality of pharmaceutical services. These guidelines have been – or are in the process of being – adopted around the world. The revised guidelines were adopted by WHO and approved by the FIP Council in 1997.

Maintaining competence throughout a career, during which new and challenging professional responsibilities will be encountered, is another fundamental ethical requirement for all health professionals. It must be a continuous, cyclical process of quality improvement by which health professionals seek to maintain and enhance their competence in both current duties and anticipated future service developments.

Effective collaboration among health professionals is key to delivering cost-effective and quality health care. In 2000, the international organizations representing the world's pharmacists, nurses and physicians unveiled a unique and powerful alliance, the World Health Professions Alliance (WHPA). The founding organizations are FIP, the International Council of Nurses, and the World Medical Association.

WHPA believes that reaching out to people in times of illness and wellness requires the resources and expertise of health professionals with diverse training and skills. Building on this belief, the international nurse, pharmacist and physician professions are strengthening their collaboration to bring about a higher quality of service to the public and patients.

A.J.M. Hoek
General Secretary and Chief Executive Officer
International Pharmaceutical Federation

---

[4] *Standards for quality of pharmacy services.* Vancouver, International Pharmaceutical Federation (FIP), 1998 (http://www.fip.org/pdf/gpp97_en.pdf, accessed 22 October 2004).

Supporting statement: European Respiratory Society

It is a great honour and a privilege for the European Respiratory Society (ERS) to express full support to this seminal WHO initiative. This project will certainly guide future worldwide strategic developments on education and training of health professionals. The current publication should be considered an important component of a coherent and well planned policy conducted by WHO to meet the challenges generated by the increasing impact of chronic conditions.

During the previous century, enormous progress was made in improving health, and therefore, life expectancy. However, the realization of further improvements and the achievement of seamless standards of care seem to be hampered by the inefficiencies in applying existing knowledge at the level of clinical practice. There is increasing awareness of the need for bridging the gap between research and delivery of health care services. This shall be achieved by following the new paradigms that guide this WHO initiative. Basic science, clinical discovery, and patient-oriented research are interdependent; they should not necessarily be considered successive steps.

This publication continues WHO efforts to update health care capacities to meet the needs of chronic conditions. The weight given to respiratory diseases could not be more timely, when the latest trends categorically position chronic respiratory disorders among the major causes of death. Facing this increase requires a good understanding of the clinical context and perfect knowledge of the local environment. Feasibility first, and success later, will come about only if these two factors are fully harmonized. In this sense, the insights of the case examples collected in this work provide a useful frame of reference for both physicians and policy-makers. Much can still be done through local initiatives to lessen the predicted rise in prevalence and impact of chronic conditions if such a change in the paradigm of delivering care is adopted on a large scale.

ERS, like other scientific societies, has the potential to effectively contribute to the transition toward the new health care landscape by increasing the emphasis on patient-oriented care, and the focus on public health issues. Our support for this WHO project is in full alignment with our mission. Additionally, the collaboration on this report has been a gratifying and enriching experience.

Founded in 1990, ERS is a non-profit, international organization committed to promoting education and research in respiratory medicine. With members from more than 90 countries worldwide, ERS is the leading forum in Europe for the exchange of knowledge between scientists and health professionals involved in respiratory medicine. The Society has a key role in establishing recommendations and guidelines to ensure the highest standards for health care delivery. Through the ERS School, we strongly support educational and training activities. ERS is also a founding member of the Forum of International Respiratory Societies (FIRS), an organization established in 2002 by leading professional societies from all over the world to promote education, research, patient care and public health in the field of respiratory medicine.

WHO should be congratulated for this initiative. It will be a privilege for ERS to further expand the partnership in this stimulating endeavour.

Walter McNicholas
President
European Respiratory Society

Supporting statement:
International Alliance of Patients' Organizations

The International Alliance of Patients' Organizations (IAPO) strongly supports WHO in addressing the issues of education and training of the health care workforce. It commends this work and, in particular, the opportunity for patients (through representation by patients' organizations) to contribute their very relevant opinions and experience, which IAPO asserts are a vital consideration in all aspects of health care and health care policy-making.

Relationships between health professionals and patients are of paramount importance to build patient-centred health care for patients with chronic conditions. Chronic conditions often continue for many years and affect all aspects of a person's life. This necessitates a shift in focus from the general characteristics of a disease to the personal needs and expectations of individuals and how they manage their condition, so that they can participate in life.

A productive relationship requires the involvement of health professionals, patients, families, carers, patients' organizations, and the wider community. Patients, as well as health professionals, must have the skills necessary to interact and work together. The benefits, in addition to patient satisfaction, will include improved health outcomes, and will counter some of the imperfections of health care systems, whether they are in the developing or developed world. Communication and partnering are key in these relationships.

Communication must include interactive dialogue between patients and health professionals, where listening is as important as speaking. Presentation of health information should consider health literacy principles. IAPO defines health literacy to include an individual's reading level, as well as language, education level, cultural background and readiness to receive health information by oral, written or pictorial means. Low health literacy affects a person's ability to make informed decisions about his or her health, and can result in ineffective treatment and rehabilitation of the patient's condition. A 1995 study in the United States found that one third of English-speaking hospital patients could not read or understand basic health materials; however, poor levels of health literacy exist in all countries.

Partnerships are vital. Working collaboratively with other health professionals, with patients and with the wider community will help to increase patient engagement, improve continuity of care, and overcome fragmentation of health care systems. Patients and health care professionals need to work more closely together, appreciating each other's expertise (e.g. a health professional is medical expert, and a patient is an expert in what the condition and treatment mean to them), and interacting to determine desired outcomes of the treatment.

Patients' organizations can play a vital role in these partnerships. Health professionals and patients' organizations should be encouraged to foster these relationships. Patients' organizations have a wealth of knowledge and experience of chronic conditions. Among the many opportunities to work collaboratively with health professionals, patients' organizations can provide support and information to patients to aid the individual in active engagement in their health care, thereby helping patients to change their behaviours, and assisting with self-management and adherence to therapies. They can provide advice to health professionals on the personal experiences and needs of patients – which should be considered in all aspects of health care – as part of evidence-based care, in the design of health professional training programmes and in the evaluation of services.

The training of health care professionals is vital for patient-centred health care, but health care systems and external activities must also be examined. Education of patients, their families, and carers is essential. At present, there are many patients worldwide who do not have sufficient knowledge to take an active part in the treatment of their condition, even if they so choose. They need to learn how to articulate their needs, how to locate and analyse health information from a variety of sources, and to know more about health care professionals, their work and available treatments and medications.

The involvement of patients and patients' organizations at every level where health care decisions are made is essential to build patient-centred health care worldwide.

Jo Harkness
Policy and External Affairs Director
International Alliance of Patients' Organizations

Executive summary

The health care workforce is one of the most important factors in the health care system. Health care providers are instrumental in stimulating, creating and maintaining health care improvement.

Around the world, the rapidly shifting balance between acute and chronic health problems is placing new and different demands on the health care workforce. There is general consensus that to provide effective health care for chronic conditions, the skills of health professionals must be expanded to meet these new complexities. This expansion does not invalidate the need for existing competencies, such as the practice of evidence-based and ethical care. Rather, it underscores the growing need for new competencies to complement existing ones.

First, the workforce needs to organize care around the patient, i.e. to adopt a patient-centred approach. Second, providers need the communication skills that enable them to collaborate with others. They need not only partner with patients, but work closely with other providers, and join with communities to improve outcomes for patients with chronic conditions. Third, the workforce needs skills to ensure that the safety and quality of patient care is continuously improved. Fourth, the workforce needs skills that assist them in monitoring patients across time, and using and sharing

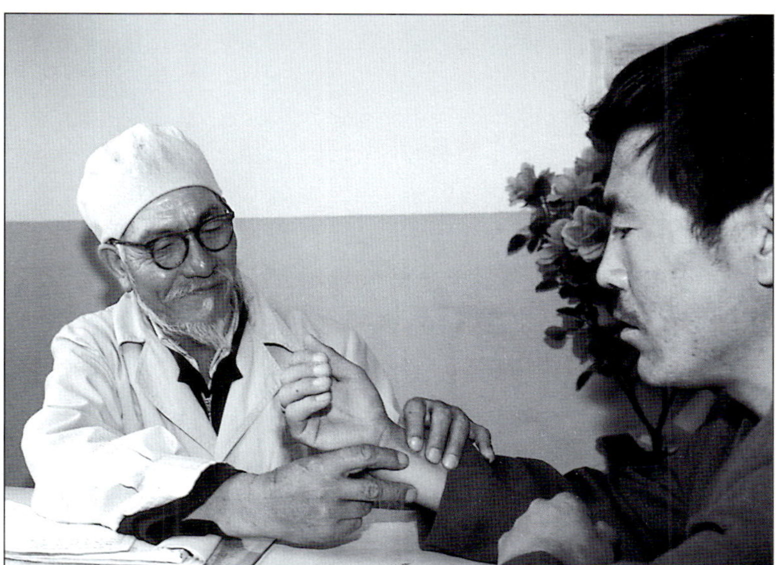

© WORLD BANK

information through available technology. Finally, the workforce needs to consider patient care and the provider's role in that care from the broadest perspective, including population-based care, the multiple levels of the health care system and the care continuum.

These abilities and skills are reflected in five basic competencies that apply to all members of the workforce caring for patients with chronic health problems:

1. patient-centred care
2. partnering
3. quality improvement
4. information and communication technology
5. public health perspective.

Within the main body of this publication, each competency is described in detail and supplemented with diverse country examples of how it has been implemented.

True educational reform of the health care workforce will not be possible without concerted and sustained efforts among decision-makers, academic leaders, and health professional bodies. This is, nonetheless, both achievable and essential.

Introduction and scope

This document is a call for the transformation of health care workforce training to better meet the needs of caring for patients with chronic conditions. For the purpose of this document, the terms *workforce* and *providers* refer to lay health workers, nurses, pharmacists, dentists, physicians and allied health professionals – all of whom provide direct care for patients with chronic conditions. *Chronic conditions* are defined as health problems that require ongoing management over a period of years or decades, and include: diabetes, heart disease, asthma, chronic obstructive pulmonary disease (COPD), cancer, HIV/AIDS, depression, and physical disabilities *(1)*. There are many other chronic conditions, but the one feature that unites them all is that they typically affect the social, psychological and economic dimensions of a person's life.

Traditional health care training is increasingly acknowledged as limited because of its fundamental focus on the diagnosis and treatment of acute medical problems (*2–4*). Although acute medical problems and illnesses will always require the attention of health care providers, a training model that is focused on managing acute symptoms is increasingly recognized as insufficient to address the concerns of the growing population of patients with chronic conditions. Training reform can expand this focus to recognize the patient from a broader perspective: from the vantage point of the patient and the patient's care continuum (i.e. from clinical prevention to palliative care).

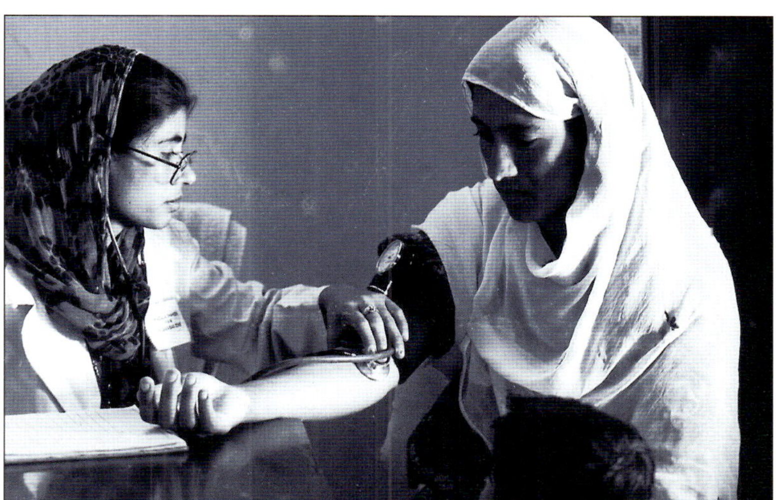

A new, expanded training model, based on a set of core competencies, could better prepare the health care workforce to care for patients with chronic conditions. Leaders who recognize the need for improvement in education and training may use this basic set of competencies as a starting point for reform. The competencies could also serve as the foundation for health care training for the 21st century. They can be implemented in a variety of established training contexts, including pre-service education, continuing education, or in-service experiences.

Today's educational and academic leaders, professional bodies, and other stakeholders invested in health care are positioned to influence rapid improvements in the training and preparation of tomorrow's cohort of health care providers. The core competencies outlined below are a guide for long overdue training reform.

Identification of competencies

Competencies are the skills, abilities, knowledge, behaviours and attitudes that are instrumental in the delivery of desired results and, consequently, of job performance. Competencies "add further definition to any job by their focus on how work is done and what work is done" *(5)*. The competencies presented here are not representative of the full range of skills that providers need for delivering health care in their respective disciplines; rather, the identified competencies are the basic, requisite and indispensable cornerstones for providing care for patients with chronic health problems that share a number of characteristics. These core competencies apply to all members of the health care workforce, irrespective of discipline.

The five core competencies were identified following a process that included document review and international expert agreement. Determination of the competencies included a review of the literature on educational reform for health care providers and health care for chronic conditions. In addition, various professional organizations' published standards and discipline-specific competencies were examined. Throughout the process, the emphasis was on the identification of competencies that addressed the needs of patients and their families. Common competencies across a variety of professional groups (including family physicians, nurses, pharmacists, dentists and allied health workers) were identified and described in a draft document. International professional councils, educational leaders, patient advocacy groups and experts in the care of patients with chronic conditions, reviewed the draft and made suggestions resulting in a final list of core competencies.

Background

The world is experiencing a rapid rise in chronic health problems to the extent that chronic conditions now account for over half of the global disease burden *(6)*. Previously, acute infectious diseases were the primary focus of the health care workforce in every country. However, during the last century, advances in medical science, technology and public health, such as immunizations, sanitation, housing and education, have contributed to a decrease in acute diseases. As a result, life expectancy has risen during this period.

Because people are living longer, they have the opportunity for extended exposure to risks that promote the development of chronic conditions. For example, unhealthy behaviours that have escalated due to aggressive marketing of tobacco, alcohol and unhealthy foods, increase the likelihood of the onset of many chronic conditions *(7)*. Physical inactivity is a significant risk factor for chronic conditions as is poverty *(1)*, which continues to affect a large percentage of the world's population and is inextricably intertwined with chronic health concerns. Public and social policies do not consistently promote health and support strategies to prevent the development of chronic problems. Clearly, the determinants of chronic conditions are complex: multifactoral and multisectoral.

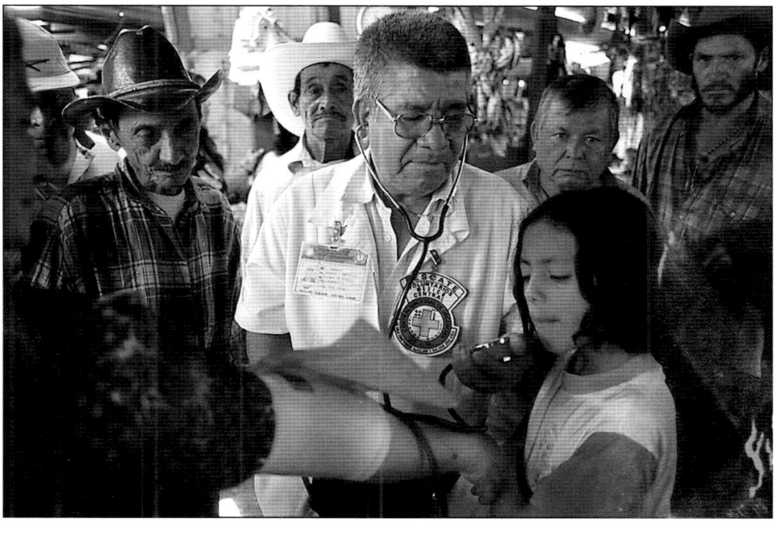

© WORLD BANK

While the world is experiencing a rapid escalation in chronic health problems, training of the health care workforce has, generally, not kept pace. Many authors have noted that the training, education, and skill set of today's health care personnel is not adequate to manage patients with chronic conditions *(1, 2, 8–11)*. Moreover, while providers currently treat patients with diabetes, asthma and heart disease as a matter of routine, they report that their preparation for coordinating care and educating patients with chronic conditions is inadequate *(12)*.

The reason for the ill-prepared workforce is straightforward: Caring for patients with chronic conditions is different from caring for patients with episodic illnesses, and the workforce is better prepared to care for the latter. Patients with chronic health problems need care that is coordinated across time and centred on their needs, values and preferences. They need

FIGURE 1. The Innovative Care for Chronic Conditions Framework *(1)*.

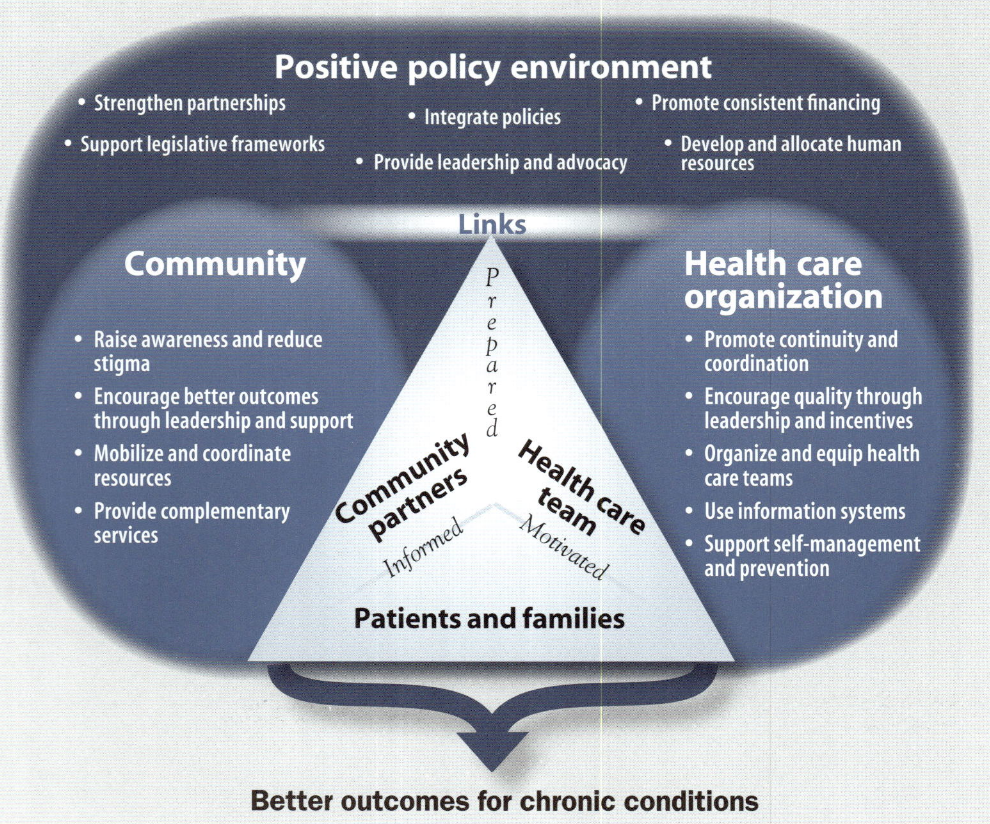

self-management skills to ensure the prevention of predictable complications, and they need providers who understand the fundamental difference between episodic illness that is identified and cured, and chronic conditions that require management across many years.

Reform in training the workforce is only one component of the more general health care system reform that is needed to improve care for patients with chronic conditions. To create a well functioning health care system, reform is necessary at multiple levels; WHO has provided a conceptual framework to address this pressing need of improving care for chronic conditions (see Figure 1). The Innovative Care for Chronic Conditions (ICCC) Framework *(1)* is an expanded, internationalized adaptation of the earlier Chronic Care Model developed by Wagner and colleagues *(13)*. The framework outlines the components necessary to improve care for patients across multiple levels of the health care system: the general policy environment, the health care organization and community, and the patient-care level. Optimally, patients and their families are the centre of the system, communities connect with health care organizations, and these relationships work best when enveloped within a policy environment that organizes the values, principles and general strategies of governments working to reduce the burden of chronic conditions.

The ICCC Framework is a starting point for overall health care system improvement. It describes the essential components necessary to improve outcomes associated with chronic conditions. However, transformation in health care organizations is impossible without transformation in the workforce that provides the care. The current document is restricted to this single topic: training reform for the workforce that cares for patients with chronic health concerns. Clearly, education and training are not the sole answers to improving care for patients; however, they are essential components of the solution.

The need for a new perspective

Health care for patients with chronic conditions requires a fundamental change in perspective from the familiar approach, which evolved out of treating acute illnesses. However, shifting from the prevailing perspective to one of planning health care over years or a lifetime is a significant challenge to the workforce and educational leaders alike. The magnitude of the challenge eases somewhat with the knowledge that chronic conditions share many common features. In fact, comparable management strategies are effective across all chronic health problems, making seemingly disparate conditions such as heart disease, diabetes, disabilities and depression, far more alike than different. Whereas biomedical treatment is dependent upon the unique features of a specific disease, the general components of health care for chronic conditions – meaning its organization and delivery, and provider disease management skills – are essentially the same. These components include: a well defined care plan, patient self-management, scheduled follow-up appointments, monitoring of outcome and adherence, and step-by-step treatment protocols *(14–20)*.

Concisely, patients with chronic conditions need health care that emerges from a longitudinal perspective with an emphasis on prevention *(21)*. Providers need vigilance regarding two types of prevention: preventing the occurrence of chronic conditions in the first place, and preventing predictable complications of chronic conditions through optimal treatment and management of chronic conditions once they have occurred. Self-management and collaboration are essential features of this care *(22)*.

Core competencies for caring for patients with chronic conditions

A reconceptualization of patient care translates into the need for a new set of workforce competencies. This expansion does not invalidate the need for existing competencies, such as the practice of evidence-based and ethical care. Rather, it underscores the growing need for new competencies to complement existing ones.

First, the workforce needs to organize care around the patient, i.e. adopt a patient-centred approach. This focus has been described as one in which the provider "tries to enter the patient's world, to see the illness through the eyes of the patient" *(23)*. Second, providers need communication skills that enable them to collaborate with others. They need not only to partner with patients, but to work closely with other providers and join with communities to improve outcomes for patients with chronic conditions. Third, the workforce needs skills to ensure that the safety and quality of patient care are continuously improved. Fourth, the workforce needs skills that assist them in monitoring patients across time, using and sharing information through available technology. Finally, the workforce needs to consider patient care and the provider's role in that care from the broadest perspective, including population-based care, multiple levels of the health care system, and the care continuum.

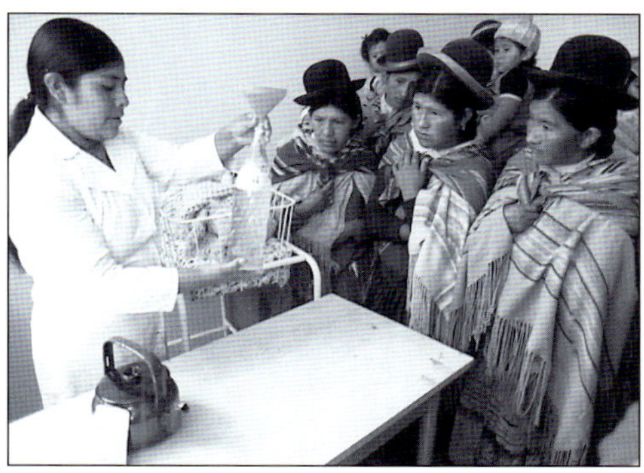

How can educational leaders and other stakeholders ensure the workforce gains adequate expertise in these new areas? A practical place to begin is to define and build consensus around a set of core competencies. This publication proposes the five basic competencies that apply to all members of the workforce caring for patients with chronic health problems, as outlined in Table 1 (see next page).

TABLE 1: CORE COMPETENCIES DESCRIBED IN THIS PUBLICATION

1. Patient-centred care
- Interviewing and communicating effectively
- Assisting changes in health-related behaviours
- Supporting self-management
- Using a proactive approach

2. Partnering
- Partnering with patients
- Partnering with other providers
- Partnering with communities

3. Quality improvement
- Measuring care delivery and outcomes
- Learning and adapting to change
- Translating evidence into practice

4. Information and communication technology
- Designing and using patient registries
- Using computer technologies
- Communicating with partners

5. Public health perspective
- Providing population-based care
- Systems thinking
- Working across the care continuum
- Working in primary health care-led systems

These core competencies have the potential to shift current thinking about providing care for patients with ongoing health problems and, in turn, to reform the training and preparation of the health care workforce. The five competencies do not replicate or preclude established core competencies (*2, 4, 24–26*). Rather, these core competencies augment existing knowledge and skills to provide better care for patients living with chronic health problems.

Core Competency 1:

Patient-centred care

A shift in training from provider-centred to patient-centred care is a competency specifically recommended by several health care disciplines and professional bodies (*2, 4, 9, 27–29*). Emphasis on this core competency alone has the potential to transform health care. Centring care upon the patients allows their values, preferences, needs and expertise to direct care for the chronic problems with which they live.

Patient-centred care is broad in scope and requires a multitude of skills of the workforce. The components of patient-centred care include:

- identifying, caring about and respecting patients' preferences, values, differences and expressed needs
- coordinating continuous and timely care
- relieving pain and suffering
- listening and communicating
- providing education and information
- sharing decision-making and management
- preventing disease, disabilities, and impairments
- promoting wellness and healthy lifestyles *(2)*.

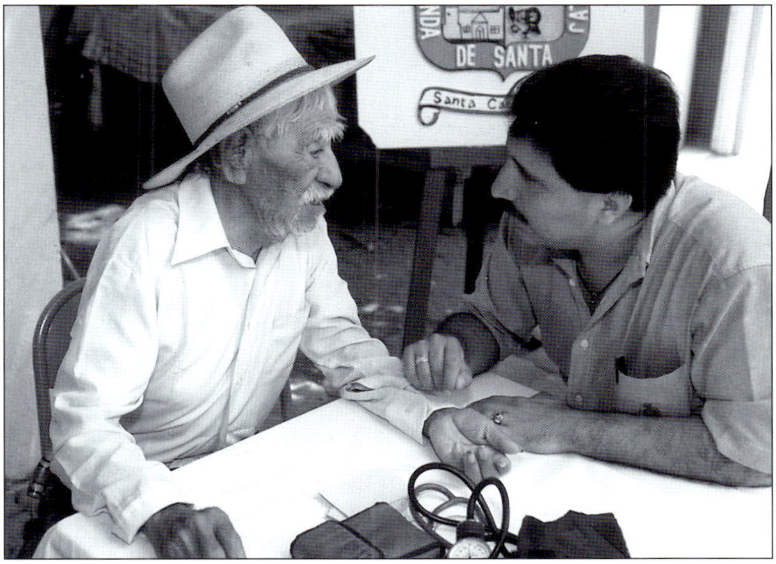

Patient-centred care

Patient-centred care improves outcomes: satisfaction with care increases and adherence to medical recommendations improves when patients are actively included (*22, 30*).

In effect, by increasing the focus on the patient, patient-centred care strengthens the role of patients in managing their health problems. From this perspective, patients and their families become experts in their own care and needs, and develop as the principal caregivers for their problems (*22, 31*). In patient-centred care, patients shift from being passive recipients of care to being active decision-makers.

1.1 Interviewing and communicating effectively

To focus care on the patient, the workforce needs communication skills that elicit information from the patient's point of view, instil confidence in the confidentiality of the interaction, and meet the patient at his or her unique level of understanding. The workforce needs to be trained to enquire comfortably about patients' concerns, emotions, social situations and behaviours *(32)*. Providers need sufficient training in interviewing, which will enable them to identify potential problems, and allow patients to express – without judgement – their values and preferences for care *(11)*. Cultural issues and the patient's ability to comprehend health information, sometimes called "health literacy level" *(3)*, are more likely to be identified during an interview that creates a supportive context and encourages questions from patients. In some cases, interpreters and/or culturally appropriate techniques will be indicated *(33)*. In other circumstances, it will be necessary to share written materials that use graphics and simple words *(34)*.

1.2 Assisting changes in health-related behaviours

Incorporating patients as active and equal partners in their care requires a workforce capable of supporting patients' efforts in changing their behaviours to improve health and to manage chronic conditions. Assisting patients to change health-related behaviours is especially important, because research on the complex determinants of health and illness increasingly points to the role of patients' daily behaviour and decision-making *(35)*. Daily decisions (e.g. eating, physical activity, taking medications, monitoring symptoms, etc.), which to varying degrees are influenced by broader social and environmental determinants, can affect the onset, delay or total prevention of associated complications *(36)*. The workforce needs a skill set that will aid patients in changing their behaviours in order to improve health and quality of life *(3)*. Although the determinants of health-related behaviours extend far beyond the confines of the health care setting, the health care workforce can influence how patients behave in their communities. They can provide patients with information about the behaviours that will improve their health, prevent chronic conditions or delay complications once a chronic condition has occurred *(11)*. Mounting evidence demonstrates that primary care physicians can assist patients in changing behaviour using a variety of proven techniques (*37, 38*). Providers can use verbal counselling strategies (e.g. eliciting comments from patients about making changes versus allowing patients to describe reasons for not changing) to increase the motivational level of patients considering health-promoting behaviours *(39)*.

1.3 Supporting self-management

Patients with chronic conditions require a variety of self-management abilities to control symptoms and minimize complications. The workforce needs to be well-versed in these skills so that they can impart them to patients without hesitation and as a matter of routine quality care. Patients will benefit from a set of cognitive and behavioural self-management skills to minimize complications or delay their onset entirely, including:

- coping skills (i.e. managing emotions related to chronic conditions)
- goal setting for specific and moderately challenging behaviours
- self-monitoring (i.e. keeping track of behaviours)
- environmental modification (i.e. creating a context to maximize success)
- self-reward (i.e. reinforcing one's behaviour with immediate, personal and desirable rewards)
- arranging social support (i.e. gaining the support of others).

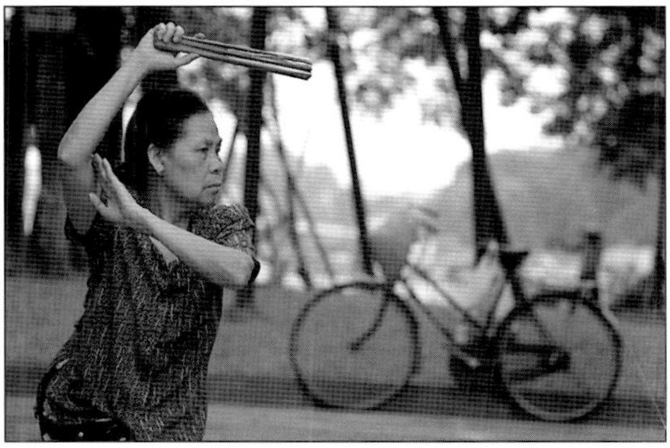

1.4 Using a proactive approach

Another component of patient-centred care is attention to and coordination of care across time. Care for chronic conditions is continuous and ongoing, and as such, the workforce must be competent in conducting, planning and ensuring that patients receive scheduled follow-up visits. During follow-up visits, the workforce can employ skills to monitor patients' response to treatment, and adherence to negotiated care plans. Patients' behavioural self-management efforts can be rewarded, problem-solving can be assisted, anticipated difficulties can be reviewed, and solid, long-term patient-provider relationships can grow.

In summary, systematic reviews show that patient-centred care results in increased adherence to care plans, reduced morbidity, and improved quality of life for patients *(40)*. A patient-centred approach to care could be especially important in low-resource contexts where the health care workforce, medications and equipment are in limited supply, and where wasted resources have a particularly adverse impact. Ultimately, the success of the health care workforce and health care organizations depends upon the extent to which they can focus care on using the patients' perspective to increase their engagement in continuing and/or adopting behaviours that best promote health and delay complications related to chronic conditions.

CASE EXAMPLES: PATIENT-CENTRED CARE

CANADA:

Supporting self-management/Using a proactive approach for COPD *(41)*

Chronic obstructive pulmonary disease is a major public health problem. Approximately 40–50% of COPD patients discharged from hospitals are readmitted during the following year, and 17% of COPD patients discharged from emergency departments require hospitalization. Innovative home-based services to support selected groups of COPD patients have shown safety, efficacy and cost-containment, but the role of case management programmes in improving health service utilization and health status in clinically stable COPD patients were inconclusive.

A multicentre randomized clinical trial conducted in seven city hospitals in Quebec, Canada, showed that a continuum of self-management

(Continues on next page…)

(Continued from previous page)

for advanced, clinically-stable COPD patients provided by trained health professionals, can significantly reduce the utilization of health care services, and improve health status.

The intervention consisted of a comprehensive patient education programme administered through weekly visits by trained health professionals over a two-month period, with monthly follow-up by telephone. The primary outcome during the 12-month follow-up period was number of hospital admissions. Secondary outcomes included emergency visits and patient health status. Patients had at least one hospitalization for COPD exacerbation in the previous year. They were elderly, not highly educated, with severe lung function impairment and significant comorbidities (cardiovascular 45%, diabetes 22%, and gastrointestinal 27%).

Hospital admissions for exacerbation of COPD were reduced by 40% in the intervention group, as compared with the control group. Hospital admissions for other health care problems, emergency room visits and unscheduled physician visits, showed significant reductions in the self-management group as well. A beneficial impact of the intervention on health-related quality of life was also observed, and maintained at 12 months.

The study showed that case management promoted continuity, communication and collaboration among the patient, the family and health care providers, and made a positive impact on outcomes. Because the approach does not require highly specialized resources, it can be easily implemented within normal practice by professionals as an integral part of the long-term care of patients with moderate to advanced COPD.

CHINA:

Supporting self-management [42]

Self-management for people with chronic disease is now widely recognized as a necessary part of treatment. The community-based Chronic Disease Self-Management Programme (CDSMP) is the most widely accepted self-management patient education programme worldwide, because it is designed to meet the needs of patients who have more than one chronic condition, and it is taught by trained lay leaders.

Noncommunicable diseases – primarily heart disease, stroke, cancer, and lung disease – were responsible for 81% of the deaths in China in 1996 and accounted for a major portion of total health care costs. Prevention and management of chronic disease is an urgent primary health problem to be addressed in Shanghai. The inability of current major health care systems to deal with chronic conditions calls for prompt policy action and new approaches to people with chronic conditions. A Chinese CDSMP, and its locally-based delivery model, were developed in Shanghai from 1999 to 2001. A randomized controlled trial with 954 participants demonstrated that the Shanghai CDSMP improved participants' health behaviour, self-efficacy and health status, and reduced the number of hospitalizations after six months. Until now, the programme has been implemented in 13 communities and six districts of Shanghai, and is being replicated in other cities.

(Case examples continue on next page. . .)

Patient-centred care

Mexico:

Reorienting care around patients [43]

The *Clínica y Hospital de Especialidades*, a small rural hospital located in the town of Nuevo Laredo, Mexico, delivers health care that reflects an organizational philosophy of "service to patients" as the determinant of quality care. Its organizational chart identifies the patient and family at the top, directly supported by hospital personnel whose purpose is to attend to human needs first, and medical needs second. Patients and visitors are greeted at the door of the hospital, where they receive information without having to seek it out. Patient rooms have a separate area for visitors.

Diagnostic and administrative technology is less noticeable throughout the *Clínica* than in many other health care organizations. A few computers are available, but charting, scheduling and record keeping are mostly with paper and pencil. Physicians' offices and laboratories are equipped with all the necessary tools to support common patient problems. If patients present concerns that require further investigation, however, they are referred to another level of care. Rather than emphasizing high technology care, the central focus of care is the patients and their families. The driving goal is "that patients should be made whole again, in all aspects of their lives."

World Health Organization:

Integrated Management of Adolescent and Adult Illness: Interviewing and communicating effectively/ Assisting changes in health-related behaviours [44]

WHO's Integrated Management of Adolescent and Adult Illness (IMAI) project is aimed at providing simplified guidelines for care of adolescents and adults by multipurpose primary-level facility health workers in low resource settings with a high prevalence of HIV/AIDS.

Because the management of chronic conditions (including HIV/AIDS) requires active participation of patients, the *IMAI General Principles of Chronic Care* are focused on equipping health care workers to provide patient-centred health care. Specifically, the guidelines and related training materials prepare health care workers to solicit patients' concerns and preferences, work in collaboration with patients to decide specific goals and treatment plans, and support patients in their daily efforts for prevention, medication adherence and self-management. Focusing on the patient in this way constitutes an important shift in current clinical practice.

Early results indicate that the '5As' approach (assess, advise, agree, assist and arrange) to patient-centred health care, which is embedded in the IMAI, is understandable and usable by primary-level health workers. Physicians, nurses and lay providers have been trained in Burkina Faso, Burundi, Ethiopia, the Sudan and Uganda.

Core Competency 2:

Partnering

Health care for chronic conditions is a complex interaction of people and other factors around the patient. To enhance care coordination and health outcomes, providers need partnering skills as a core competency. This includes the ability to partner with patients, and to join with patients' families. Other health care providers are also part of the interaction: those who care for the patient across time, in different settings, from different disciplines and for different comorbid health concerns.

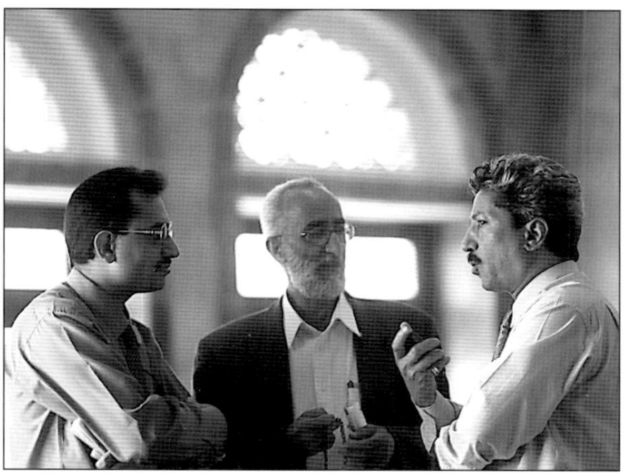

© WORLD BANK

When health problems are chronic, coordination of care becomes a high priority. Care must be organized and coordinated over time, among providers and across settings. In addition, the health care workforce will benefit patients by partnering with and understanding the communities in which patients live and make daily decisions about their health and chronic condition management. Patients' needs do not always match with services available in one institution. Partnerships have the potential to address problems that a single entity, or health worker, cannot resolve alone *(45)*.

Communication is the essential element in successful partnering, but it involves more than a friendly personality. Communication is comprised of a set of skills that can be taught, learned and maintained *(46)*. A basic set of communication skills will prepare the workforce to collaborate effectively with others – patients, providers, and/or communities. These skills include the ability to:

- negotiate
- share decisions
- collectively solve problems
- establish goals

Partnering

- implement action
- identify strengths and weaknesses
- clarify roles and responsibilities
- evaluate progress.

The application of these general partnering skills with patients, other providers and communities follows.

2.1 Partnering with patients

"Health care is relationship-centred *(4)*." Providers need communication skills that allow them to share power and involve patients in all aspects of health care decision-making. This concept overlaps somewhat with the competency of patient-centred care, and a shift toward equality of power and responsibility between patients and providers has been advocated by some for decades *(47)*. Today, empirical evidence supports an egalitarian relationship: shared patient-provider power and improved clinical outcomes are correlated *(48)*. Sharing power with patients creates an atmosphere in which patients mutually participate in care. When information about treatment, goals and expected outcomes is shared with patients, they are prepared to take greater responsibility *(49)*.

2.2 Partnering with other providers

The ability to work with other health care providers, both within and across professional disciplines, is an important area of reform identified by a number of professional bodies (*2, 4, 8, 25, 27, 50, 51*). When health care providers collaborate and work together, outcomes for patients with chronic conditions improve (*13, 22, 52–57*).

To be competent in collaborating with each other, providers need skills that promote cooperation, communication and the integration of care. To do this, the health care workforce must work interdependently, while demonstrating mutual respect, trust, support and appreciation of each discipline's unique contribution *(4)*. Training in basic group skills, such as problem identification, negotiation and conflict resolution, future planning, and role and responsibility identification, is necessary for adequate functioning *(2)*.

2.3 Partnering with communities

Creating and maintaining partnerships with communities is a competency recommended by several groups (*4, 24, 58*). Health care for patients with chronic conditions is improved when there are links between health care organizations, patients and their families, and community resources *(22)*. Community partners can be as diverse as employers, academic institutions, civil society groups, media representatives, government bodies, patient advocacy groups and faith-based organizations. The health care workforce needs partnering skills that promote the development of patient referral pathways between the health care setting and community organizations. Communication skills that nurture and maintain these partnerships are also crucial.

Developing the competency to partner with the community will help to redistribute responsibility between the health care system, and the neighbourhoods and villages in which patients spend the majority of their time. In fact, the Pew Commission *(4)* suggests that health care professionals "embrace individuals, families, *and communities* as full and equal partners in health care decisions and provide them with the information they need to consider available alternatives and make informed choices." The ICCC Framework (see Figure 1) identifies community partners as equally important as the patient (and his/her family) and the health care workforce. This triad makes up the centrepiece of the ICCC Framework's internationally relevant model of health care for chronic conditions.

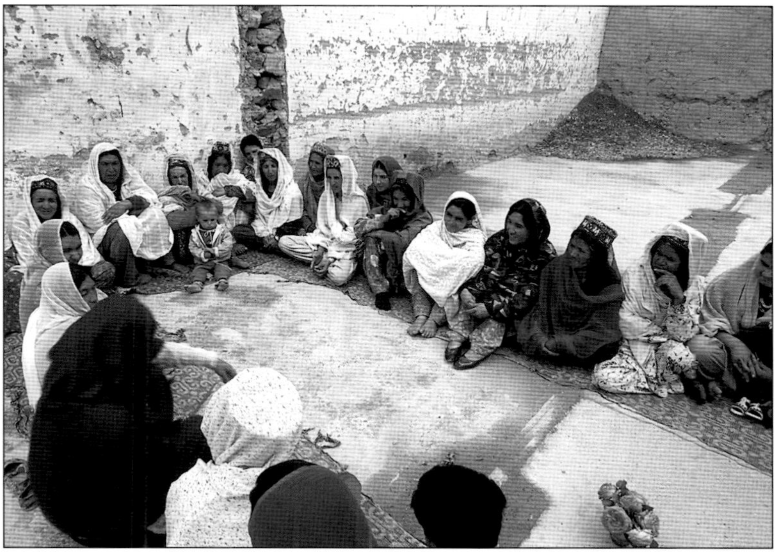

Partnering

CASE EXAMPLES: PARTNERING

Australia:

Partnering with other providers and communities [59]

The life expectancy of Australian Aborigines is 20 years less than the rest of the Australian population. Sixty-six percent of the premature deaths are due to chronic conditions, such as diabetes, hypertension and renal disease. These conditions are related in that they share risk factors and markers, are easily and cheaply diagnosed, and respond to standard treatments.

The Australian Chronic Disease Outreach Programme on the Tiwi Islands serves as a model of best practices to other communities and countries. Critical components of the programme include:

- eliciting the concerns of the community when setting priorities;
- developing partnerships with remotely located health care teams (providing them with education and information systems);
- performing simple diagnostic tests, using health care workers to interpret them (this allows for immediate feedback and education of the patient);
- treating according to evidence-based guidelines, using medications in a sequence of increasing intensity.

Positive clinical outcomes

- blood pressure is monitored in 75% of people with previously unrecognized hypertension;
- haemoglobin A1C is tested in 91% of people with diabetes;
- savings in dialysis avoided (mean treatment time 2.1 years) AUD$ 700 000 to AUD$ 3.1 million;
- hospitalizations have declined.

Programme successes

- The Federal Government now allows health care workers to bill for their services on behalf of their clinic.
- The information and communications technology (ICT) systems for primary care are provided free of charge to all communities by the Federal Government.
- Aboriginal communities access medicines through federally-funded pharmaceutical benefits.
- Screening and treatment guidelines are officially incorporated in the protocols of primary care in each region and in national guidelines.

(Case examples continue on next page...)

FINLAND:

Partnering with patients, other providers, and communities [60]

The Diabetes Programme for Pharmacies (DPP) is a supplementary programme under the Development Programme for the Prevention and Care of Diabetes (DEHKO). DEHKO has been nationally organized by the Finnish Diabetes Association to address the increase in type 2 diabetes. Pharmacies collaborate with other health care providers and patient groups to establish best practices. Such practices involve participating pharmacies hosting a contact person to liase between the Association of Finnish Pharmacies and the pharmacy. Tasks include: maintaining internal diabetes training within pharmacies, the provision of an annual report, and standardized local-level follow-up on a yearly basis. Because patients with diabetes visit pharmacies approximately six times a year, these visits can be crucial opportunities in disease supervision with regards to obtaining information on the correct usage of medication, as well as being guided in self-management techniques. DPP aims to promote more effective treatment for type 2 diabetes by emphasizing prevention of the disease, and making diabetes an issue for pharmacies to address daily.

MOROCCO:

Partnering with other providers for the integrated management of respiratory diseases [61]

The WHO Practical Approach to Lung Health (PAL) programme is a coordinated strategy for the management of respiratory diseases that relies on the standardization of care practices and coordination between different levels of care. Four diseases are the primary focus of the PAL strategy: tuberculosis, acute respiratory infections, asthma and COPD.

Since its inception in 1997, the PAL programme has developed guidelines, study protocols, training and other materials for their implementation in low- and middle-income countries.

Morocco figures prominently in the list of early adopters of the PAL approach as a way of extending the outstanding success of its national tuberculosis programme to other respiratory conditions. With a good partnership between the public and private sectors, Morocco exhibits its tuberculosis detection and treatment rates of 90%, with low prevalence of primary drug and multi-drug resistance.

PAL guidelines adapted to the country context were introduced in primary care centres with a focus on respiratory symptoms rather than on diseases. They proved to be useful for general practitioners and nurses through the increased standardization of patient management, and

(Continues on next page. . .)

Partnering

(Continued from previous page)

the rationalization of the prescription process. Furthermore, clear criteria for referral helped to allocate resources to patients in a more cost-efficient way.

At the secondary health care level, the Moroccan PAL strategy defines care paths that ensure the adequate continuum of care with a special emphasis on chronic respiratory conditions. The guidelines also include indicators for the evaluation of referrals. The country government has additionally supported the development of an information system for data collection and analysis.

South Africa:

Partnering with other providers and communities [62]

Alexandra Health Centre and University provides free health care, medications and education. Services include a 24-hour casualty and maternity unit, chronic disease service, antenatal/gynaecological/family planning clinic, outreach services/satellite clinics, and outpatient/labour unit.

Providers and patients routinely face poverty and violence in this community, and supportive services are constantly under development. Collaborative attempts to address the serious concerns in the community have resulted in 'Meals on Wheels' services, programmes for child abuse, and programmes for male health and sexually transmitted infections. Although collaborative practice is a necessity for the providers, the extended collaboration with the community has provided a model of integrated health service delivery that has persisted over seven decades.

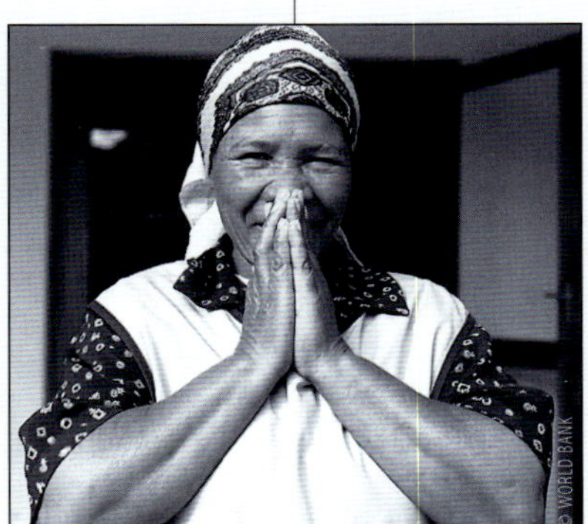

Nurses and nurse practitioners provide the majority of assessments, examinations, and evaluations to over 1000 patients daily. Consultation, back-up, and referral are available through collaboration with physicians and medical students. Further collaboration occurs with the pharmacist and pharmacy students, physical therapists, occupational therapists, social workers and volunteers.

The development of partnerships, collaboration and teamwork are the basis of the care provided at the centre. Trust is the key element to ongoing quality collaborative practice.

Positive outcomes

- shared expertise and knowledge for improved health care delivery
- balanced responsibility among partners and increased uniformity of care
- expanded health care services to the population.

Core Competency 3:

Quality improvement

Quality improvement is a competency recommended by several health-related professional bodies *(2, 4, 25, 27, 50, 58, 63)*. It is a broad concept, but continuous quality improvement captures an approach and attitude towards health care that is essential in the context of chronic condit ons. In general, quality improvement requires the health care workforce to be clear about the outcomes they are working towards; to know which changes would lead to improvements; and to know how to evaluate their efforts *(64)*. In addition, it requires them to translate evidence from their own improvement efforts, and those of others, into practice.

Patient safety and efficiency of service delivery are embedded in the quality improvement competency. Errors, waste and inefficiencies in health care are well documented *(11)*. However, a growing body of literature describes quality improvement methods as effective in mitigating errors, reducing waste, increasing efficiency and minimizing delays in diagnosis and treatment *(65–67)*. A workforce of health care providers needs to possess the abilities outlined herein to ensure quality improvement.

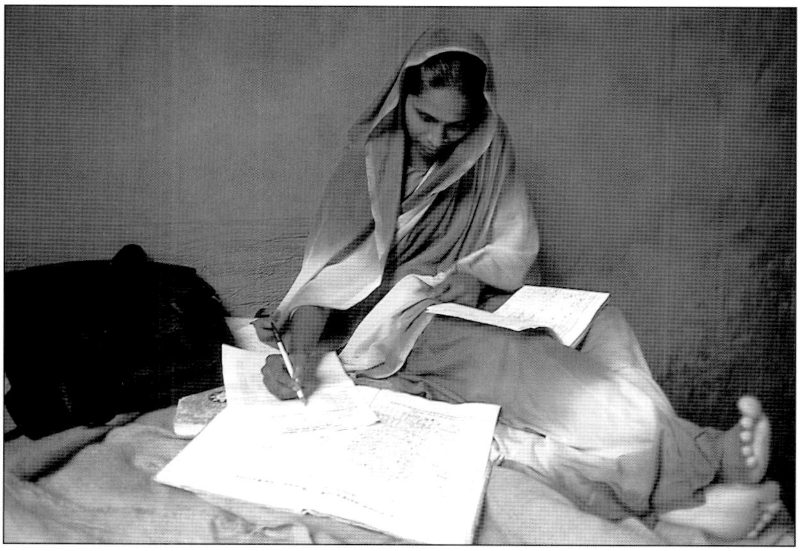

© WORLD BANK

3.1 Measuring care delivery and outcomes

A number of specific skills are necessary to enable the workforce to apply quality improvement approaches in their work. They need the ability to design and test interventions with the goal of improving quality, safety and efficiency. The workforce also needs the ability to measure quality in terms of the structure, process, and outcomes of care. Quality improvement skills include knowing how to assess current practices and compare them to new practices that might produce better outcomes. The workforce needs to be able to identify errors in care and apply basic safety design principles such as standardization and simplification of processes to reduce hazards *(11, 50, 68)*.

3.2 Learning and adapting to change

Continuous quality improvement requires an attitudinal element, in addition to the basic measurement skills outlined above. The ability to accept change and strive continuously to make things better for patients may be an equally important aspect of this core competency. Rapid advances in scientific knowledge, technology, population demographics and health care systems make it clear that mastering today's content areas in health care will not adequately prepare the workforce for managing tomorrow's changing health care problems.

The health care workforce not only needs to be capable of accepting change and managing it, but also to be prepared to embrace change and capitalize upon it. The success of health care systems depends on a flexible, innovative and adaptive workforce *(4, 8, 69)*. All members of the workforce must have these competencies, or risk losing autonomy and influence.

3.3 Translating evidence into practice

The concept of evidence is not limited to randomized clinical trials. This competency includes the ability to integrate all sources of knowledge and evidence into practice. Randomized clinical trials are part of this evidence, but clinician experience and patient circumstances should also be incorporated *(2)*. Evidence from quality improvement efforts is also included here. Health care workers should understand the value and rationale behind translating evidence into practice. They need to have the skills to formulate questions, know where and how to find relevant answers, and integrate this information into patient care.

CASE EXAMPLES: QUALITY IMPROVEMENT

MEXICO:

Measuring care delivery and outcomes/ Learning and adapting to change [70]

The monitoring system for quality of care in Mexico indicated that in 2000, only 34% of persons with diabetes who were receiving care were reported to have adequate glycemic control. As a result, in 2001, diabetes was added as a health priority, and a collaborative initiative between the Pan American Health Organization (PAHO)/ WHO and the Secretary of Health of Mexico (offices of Diabetes Action Programme from the Sub-Secretary of Disease Prevention and Control and the Sub-Secretary for Quality and Innovation). The Veracruz Initiative for Diabetes Awareness Project is the pilot phase of this initiative and is being conducted in five primary care centres. The coverage of the initiative is planned to expand nationally as part of a much larger service improvement campaign called "The Crusade for Quality Improvement".

A health technology assessment was conducted to identify the gaps in current health care practices for chronic conditions compared to best practice evidence, based on the Chronic Care Model, and to decide on priorities for a quality improvement package for change.

The goals of the project are to:

- improve capacity and knowledge of diabetes care among providers
- develop patient support groups
- improve glycemic control
- prevent diabetic complications.

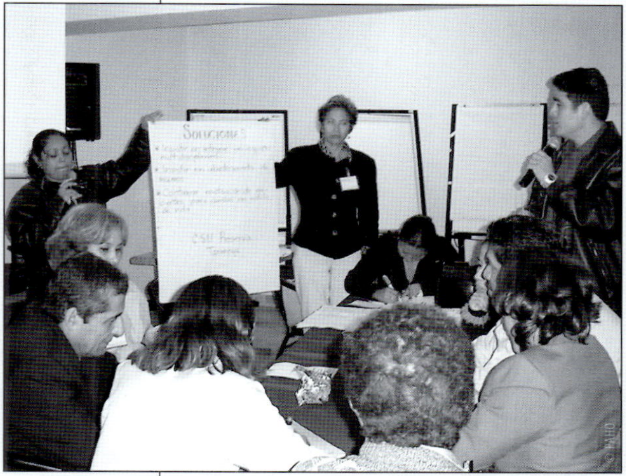

Outcomes of the pilot project:

- organization of collective medical visits for diabetic clubs
- use of lay health promoters to carry out diabetes education
- in-service training of primary care providers on diabetes management.

(Case examples continue on next page. . .)

Oman:

Measuring care delivery and outcomes/ Learning and adapting to change [71,72]

Oman is a relatively small country, 92% of which is desert, with a population of 2.5 million. In 1970, morbidity and mortality rates were high, and major communicable and infectious diseases were prevalent; the average life expectancy was 49 years. Health care services included two small hospitals and nine clinics.

Between 1970 and 2000, Oman underwent a quality improvement redesign of its health care system, and made a commitment to providing its citizens and residents with quality health care. The following strategies were initiated:

- The Ministry of Health assessed the health-related human resource requirements, including the availability and training needs of personnel.
- Policy analysis and recommendations were made to align policies to be supportive of health initiatives.
- Research studies, planning exercises, and evaluations of the recommendations were undertaken.

Positive outcomes

- in 2001, the Oman health system ranked first among 191 WHO Member States for efficiency; eighth for overall health system performance;
- in 2002, there were 48 hospitals and 128 health centres;
- a decentralized primary health care system was developed;
- programmes for health promotion, disease prevention, treatment, data collection/evaluation/feedback, and safety were coordinated, and intersectoral collaboration was established.

(Case examples continue on next page. . .)

The Netherlands, Poland and the United States

Translating evidence into practice for COPD (73,74)

The Global Initiative for Chronic Obstructive Lung Disease report states that because of its widespread use and reproducibility, spirometry is the test of choice for determining airflow limitation. Performing a spirometry test is an easy, inexpensive way to detect COPD in a preclinical phase, providing health professionals and patients with an opportunity to avert further progression of the disease.

Nonetheless, spirometry is not frequently performed in primary care settings, despite the fact that most commercially available spirometers incorporate quality control software that checks for the correct administration of the test.

Several experiences illustrate the benefits of adopting a COPD screening strategy using spirometry:

- In a pilot programme in the Netherlands, spirometry was performed on 651 smokers in two semi-rural general practice offices. The researchers reported that a new COPD case per week was identified, if at least one adult smoker was tested every day.
- In Poland, a prevention programme carried out since 2001 included the performance of spirometry in outpatient facilities. Twenty-five percent of the 11 000 tested patients with a tobacco use history presented airflow limitations compatible with early COPD stage. A smoking cessation programme was implemented in these patients. One year later, airflow limitation was found in only 50% of these patients. Smoking cessation rate was significantly higher in those patients who had initially presented abnormal spirometry results showing moderate or severe airflow limitation.
- A COPD case-finding programme in the state of Vermont in the United States found that participation by health workers in one-hour workshops could be sufficient for making a shift in some medical practices towards a greater adoption of spirometry for regular screening and diagnosis.

A worldwide comprehensive action plan to achieve extensive use of high quality forced spirometry in primary care is clearly a priority to improve patients' health management.

(Case examples continue on next page...)

Quality improvement

RUSSIAN FEDERATION:

Learning and adapting to change/Translating evidence into practice [75]

Tula Oblast in the Russian Federation is an industrial town in which many residents previously received health care through factory-based clinics. A number of factories closed, leaving patients without access to services. Cardiovascular disease is a leading cause of death in Tula Oblast, accounting for 55% of adult mortality. Hypertension prevalence is estimated at 27%, and is considered a primary contributor to this mortality rate.

To address this challenge, in 1998, the United States Agency for International Development's Global Quality Assurance Project, together with the Central Public Health Research Institute of the Russian Ministry of Health and the Tula Oblast Health Authority, embarked on improving care for patients with hypertension, under the Health Committee of the America-Russia Joint Commission for Economic and Technological Cooperation. Five health care facilities, each with a multidisciplinary team of staff responsible for all clinical functions, were involved in the decision-making and planning of the project.

Goals included:

- developing evidence-based guidelines for hypertension care at the primary care level
- changing the delivery of care for hypertension to reflect the new guidelines
- promoting healthy behaviours to prevent the complications of hypertension
- reallocation of financial and human resources to facilitate implementation of these services.

Positive outcomes

- seven-fold increase in number of patients managed at primary care level
- 70% success rate in controlling hypertension
- 85% reduction in admissions for hypertension
- net savings for overall hypertension care costs of 23%.

This quality improvement project was then expanded Oblast-wide during Phase II (2000–2002) to all 289 general practitioner practices covering the whole population of Tula Oblast, and Phase III (national scale up) was launched in December 2002.

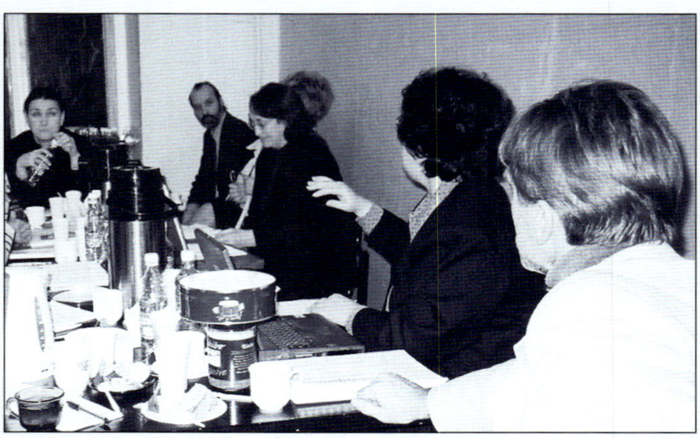

© RASHAD MASSOUD

Core Competency 4:

Information and communication technology

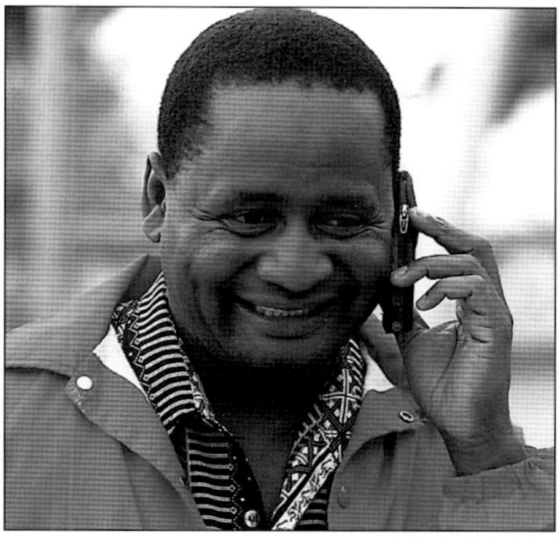
© WORLD BANK

This core competency calls for the workforce to have the skills needed to use information and communication technologies to support patient care. Information systems – from paper and pencil records to sophisticated electronic databases – are essential for organizing and monitoring patients' responses to treatments and outcomes. Communication systems allow the exchange of timely patient information with other providers, who may be in other settings. Several professional bodies have recommended that the health care workforce be capable of using information and communication systems to improve care for patients *(2, 4, 39, 76)*.

4.1 Designing and using patient registries

Information technology is commanding an increasingly important role in the health care arena. For example, some health care systems have electronic patient registries that signal and update the workforce about care plans, remind them of outreach efforts, and help to monitor patients' responses to treatment. However, information systems and patient registries do not have to be expensive. A system can be as simple as a paper and pencil-based record of patients with chronic conditions, including pertinent markers about their care. Simple information systems, if designed properly, can serve the same basic functions as sophisticated systems by monitoring the incidence and prevalence of conditions in the clinical population, monitoring individual patients' treatment and outcomes, and reminding providers about care plans.

The concept underlying this core competency is to use information systems, regardless of how plentiful the resources or advanced the technology might be, to enhance the care of patients with chronic conditions.

4.2 Using computer technologies

The use of computer technologies in health care is widespread, even in the poorest health care systems *(77)*. The so-called "digital divide" is shrinking as developing countries increasingly have access to personal digital assistants, satellite technology (instead of relying on land lines), and global networks of providers (see Figure 2). Through these advances, information and evidence about health care can be shared, expertise of scarce specialists can be pooled, and care for patients can be integrated.

To leverage available technology, the health care workforce needs a number of basic skills recommended as necessary abilities *(2)*:

- using word-processing and data analysis software
- searching online and internal databases
- retrieving and managing data

FIGURE 2. Projected Internet use in Africa (millions of users, 1995–2005)

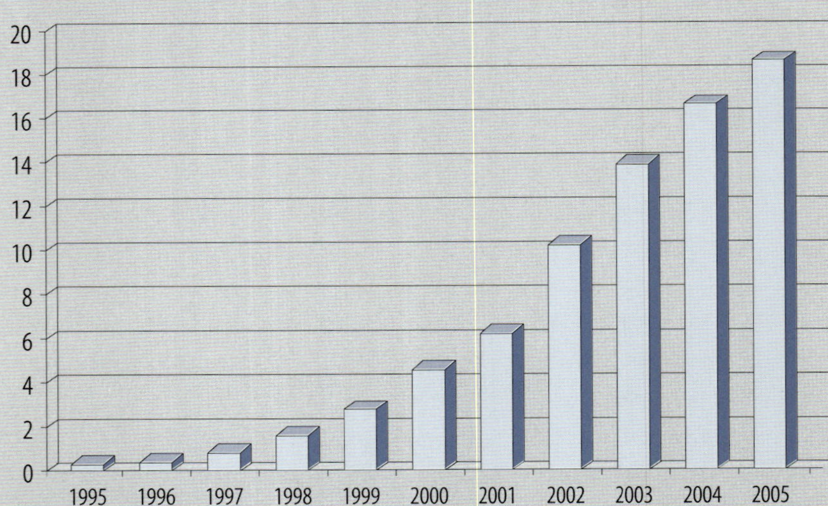

Source: International Telecommunications Union, 1 April 2004, http://www.itu.int/ITU-D/afr/statistics/projections.htm

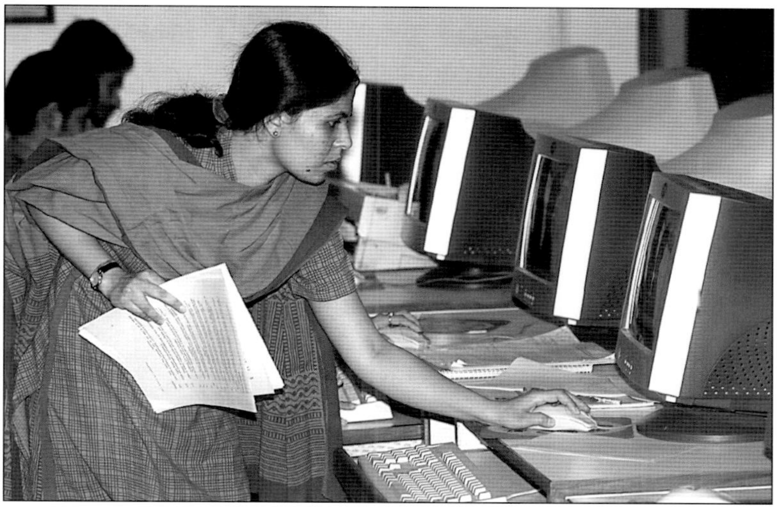

© WHO

- being aware of data security systems related to the use of patient information.

In addition, these basic skills can be used to enhance the knowledge base of the workforce by allowing them to participate in Internet-supported distance learning and continuing education opportunities. As computer technologies become increasingly available in developing countries, these competencies will become progressively more essential for providers.

4.3 Communicating with partners

Communication technology has created a variety of ways in which the health care workforce can communicate with patients, other providers, and community partners. For example, mobile phone use has increased so dramatically that in Africa the subscription rate for new mobile devices is two times that for fixed-line telephones *(78)*. The potential to use mobile phone text-messaging technology to remind patients about appointments, medication refills, or test results, is virtually untapped. Moreover, global Internet use is expanding to the extent that there are more than 605 million users worldwide *(78)*. This suggests that the workforce can increasingly communicate with partners via e-mail, and develop websites for their patients with chronic conditions. Advances in communication technologies do not render more traditional communication avenues ineffective – the workforce can continue to provide general health information to their patients and community partners using available media, such as television and newspapers.

CASE EXAMPLES: INFORMATION AND COMMUNICATIONS TECHNOLOGY

CANADA:

Communicating with partners [79]

A telehealth distance learning programme for mental health care was recently implemented and evaluated in a remote, rural region of Atlantic Canada. Urban mental health specialists provided training and support via satellite videoconferencing and Internet, print and video resources to a range of rural health and community providers. The rural participants represented diverse professions including family medicine, nursing, physiotherapy, school guidance counselling and teaching.

A total of 12 video-satellite conferences were held over a 14-month period. The specific topics were developed in response to a baseline needs survey, although the content was revised in accordance with local needs. For example, following an unusually high number of deaths in the community, two conferences were developed on managing death and bereavement. Other topics included depression, sexual abuse and coping with stress and burnout.

Evaluation indicated that participants increased their knowledge and skills as a result of the programme. Their knowledge of the roles and expertise of other professional disciplines also increased, as did their cross-disciplinary connections and referrals. These results suggest that telehealth technology can be used to facilitate training and promote interdisciplinary collaboration in rural settings.

INDIA:

Designing and using patient registries/Using computer technologies [80]

Information and communication technology has been introduced and taken shape in various ways in India. Three illustrative examples are described here.

In 2001, an interactive web site for the general public was designed by a panel of doctors in New Delhi to provide patients with chronic conditions a place to learn about their conditions and post their questions. The web site editor-in-chief says they receive approximately 65–100 questions per day from all over India and neighbouring countries.

The Health Information Network India project was initiated by a broad partnership of some 40 members comprised of United Nations agencies, nongovernmental organizations, technical experts, national and state government departments, research and health service facilities, and the private sector, to address the problem of the health-related information gap. The project was piloted in primary and community health centres in the states of Karnataka and Orissa, and supported the tuberculosis control and tobacco control programmes in research institu-

(Continued on next page. . .)

(Continued from previous page)

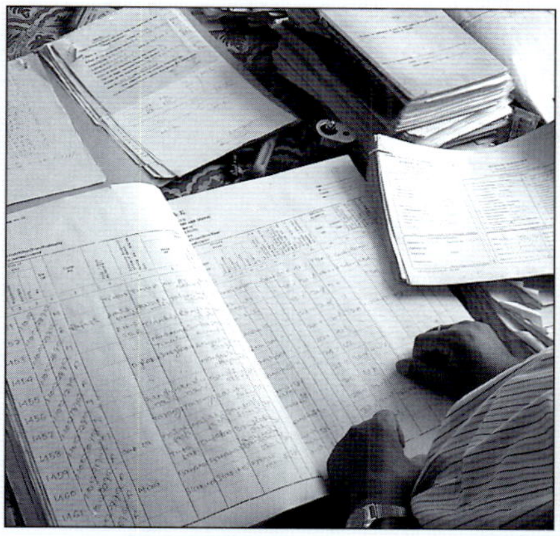

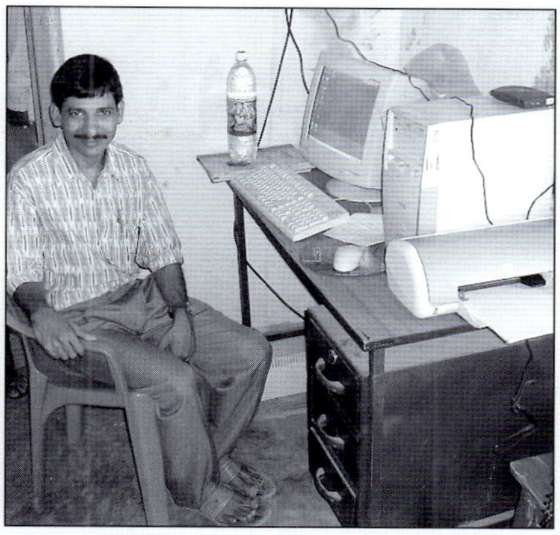

Above: The office recording system before... ...and after

tions in Mumbai, Chennai, Bangalore and Delhi. Computers were upgraded, networks and Internet connections established, and e-faxing, hand-held computers and e-consultations introduced.

Both the government and the private sector have invested in telemedicine projects with the help of the Indian Space Research Organization, which designated a domestic satellite solely for that purpose. As a result, some 20 clinics have been linked to the network, allowing for patient consultations, transmission of live surgical demonstrations and educational training.

UGANDA:

Communicating with partners [81]

The health status of Uganda's population is among the poorest worldwide because of various social, economic, environmental and infrastructural factors. The Ministry of Health has limited human and financial resources with which to address the many health care demands, and is critically aware of the need to minimize inefficiencies. The Uganda Health Information Network was created as part of the Health Sector Strategic Plan (2000/1–2004/5) to assist in the delivery of a basic health care package and national health information.

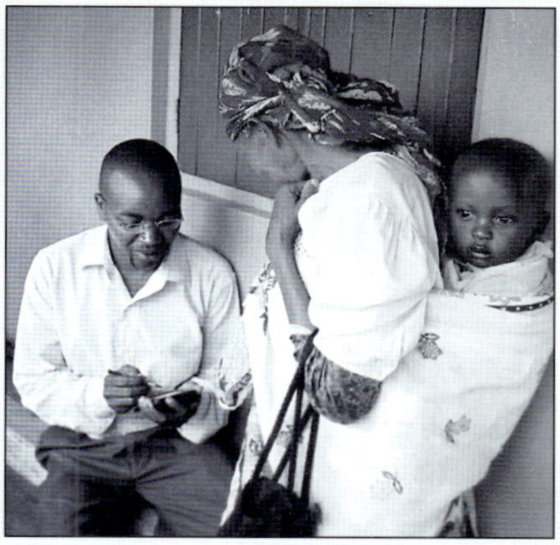

(Continued on next page...)

Information and communication technology

(Continued from previous page)

By the year 2005, providers and researchers working in 214 subdistricts, 56 districts, and referral hospitals will be connected with national level institutions using hand-held computers connected to a cellular telephone network. The network is being tested in the Mbale and Rakai districts to facilitate data collection, share new research and continuing medical education materials, and disseminate treatment guidelines. The initial implementation will determine the support and training requirements, the ongoing cost and maintenance, and the establishment of protocols for optimal functioning of the system.

The United States

Using computer technologies/Communicating with partners [82]

There is a general consensus that only a tiny fraction of the current information and communications technology developments are being used to efficiently support the process of health care.

The work carried out by the Department of Veterans Affairs Medical Centre in Boston, the United States, illustrates this point. Using existing telephone lines, the centre designed and implemented a fully automated system to monitor, educate and counsel COPD patients in the course of automated scheduled encounters in their homes.

These systems, known as "telephone-linked care", ask questions similar to those of a regular office visit, but are answered by the patient pressing the telephone keypad. The responses are then used to provide feedback to the patient. Telephone-linked care systems have been applied to the management of chronic diseases and disabilities to improve educational interventions, and to support carers. They are well accepted by both patients and health care providers, who find that they are easy to use and useful.

In the Boston experience, the goal was to detect a deteriorating condition in the patient as early as possible, to improve his/her skills in self-management and increase adherence to treatment regimes. The solution was not intended to replace conventional health care, but to complement it.

Core Competency 5:

Public health perspective

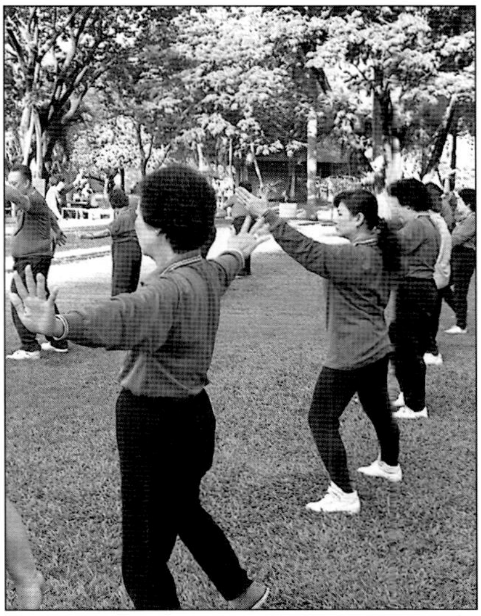

© WHO

This core competency may pose difficulties to some of the health care workforce, in that they may struggle to reconcile an abstract conceptualization of "public health" with the daily pressures and responsibilities of caring for patients' pressing needs and concerns. Nonetheless, improved common understanding between public health practitioners and the health care workforce – who traditionally approach health issues from different perspectives – will yield improved outcomes on all sides. For this to happen, however, public health must be seen as everyone's responsibility *(83)*, and the health care workforce must be engaged in the full range of advocacy, disease prevention and health promotion activities relevant to the population served.

5.1 Providing population-based care

Public health has been defined as "the science and art of preventing disease, prolonging life, and promoting health through the organized efforts of society" *(84)*. As such, thinking from a public health perspective moves the workforce from caring for one patient at a time, to planning care for populations of patients. *Population* as it is used in this context, refers to patients associated with a particular provider, clinic or health care system. This is one way in which population-based care differs from traditional, individual patient care *(85)*. A population approach does not detract from individual needs, but adds another dimension, as individuals benefit from the information developed for the populations to which they belong *(86)*. Considerations of cost-effectiveness also increase, in that patients with a

Public health perspective

specific chronic condition are prioritized so that interventions are targeted toward those members most likely to benefit *(87)*. Approaching care from a population perspective assists the workforce in balancing the value and quality of care with its costs.

To provide population-based care, the workforce needs skills to evaluate the health needs of their populations. The workforce also needs skills for implementing and evaluating evidence-based interventions in the population, with the goal of reducing risk or delaying complications in specified groups. Skills to manage populations of patients include innovative strategies for delivering care to patients who have similar needs. For example, visits provided in "group appointments" or "group consultations" – where several patients attend together – can be efficient and effective. Participants report high satisfaction with care, greater adherence with prevention activities, and less use of health care services, as compared to patients who do not participate in group medical visits *(88)*. Follow-up visits for specific populations can be provided in innovative ways and do not have to be face-to-face; where feasible, telephone calls can be used to successfully monitor patient status *(89, 90)*. Finally, the workforce needs skills that enable them to measure outcomes for *all* patients, thus avoiding the trap of focusing solely on the individual patients who present at the clinic.

Providing population-based care also implies that the health care workforce must be able to move outside formal health care settings, to work with and for the communities of their defined population. This includes involving community members as active partners in health promotion, and advocating – directly and indirectly – for disease prevention and risk reduction *(91)*. Health care providers are typically viewed as credible role models within their communities and, as such, they can influence attitudes and health behaviours, such as healthy eating, physical activity and tobacco use.

5.2 Systems thinking

Systems thinking is closely related to a public health perspective, and especially important to health care *(92)*. Whereas traditional forms of analysis isolate smaller and smaller parts of the system being studied, system-related analysis takes into account large numbers of interactions. This sometimes results in strikingly different conclusions than those generated by traditional forms of analysis, especially when what is being studied is dynamic, complex or has a great deal of feedback from other sources – such as a typical health care system *(93)*.

Health care has been described as being comprised of a series of systems which, in turn, are embedded in other, broader systems *(94)*. As such, the health care system can be divided into multiple levels: micro- or patient level, meso- or health care organization and community level, and macro- or policy level. The workforce must at least be aware of these levels, must understand how they relate to each other and, ideally, must be active in advancing public policies that affect the healthcare system *(4)*. More advanced mastery of this competency involves using systems thinking to lead innovation and change in health care systems *(92)*.

5.3 Working across the care continuum

A public health perspective emphasizes the entire care continuum, from clinical prevention to palliative care. As such, it serves the needs of the population, who require different interventions at different time points. First and importantly, the population needs preventive services, to avoid or delay the onset of chronic conditions. Every health care interaction is an opportunity for prevention, and most chronic conditions are preventable. When a condition develops, patients need evidence-based interventions and self-management support to prevent complications and disability. Patients with chronic conditions might eventually require palliative services and, ultimately, hospice care. A health care workforce that conceptualizes care from the perspective of the entire care continuum can deliver care in a more optimal way, and better meet the needs of patients with chronic conditions as well as the broader populations for which they are responsible.

5.4 Working in primary health care-led systems

In developing countries, chronic conditions present mainly at the primary health care level and need to be handled principally in these settings. To be effective across all contexts, however, primary health care must operate close to the community it serves *(95)*, including close coordination with and referral to speciality or tertiary care services, as needed.

To work in a primary health care-led system, the workforce must be able to operate effectively as a clinical team, and must have good communication skills to assure continuity of care for patients. As such, this competency is reinforced by other core competencies, such as *partnering*.

There is no single blueprint for organizing primary health care-led systems. Rather, the unique characteristics of each country should determine how primary care principles are applied in practice. Nonetheless, the shift towards primary health care-led systems implies that the workforce – in all countries – should embody its core principles *(96)*:

- universal access to care based on need
- commitment to health equity as part of social justice
- community participation in defining and implementing health agendas
- intersectoral approaches to health.

CASE EXAMPLES: PUBLIC HEALTH PERSPECTIVE

AUSTRALIA:

Systems thinking/Working across the care continuum [97,98]

Intersectoral collaboration is essential to the promotion of health because it is determined to some degree by the social, political, physical and economic factors that lie outside the biomedical sphere of influence. Moreover, "health cannot be attained by the health sector alone" *(97)*. In spite of this strategy being widely acknowledged among health professionals as an important component of health promotion, a challenge exists in having sectors other than health recognize and appreciate the impact of their products and work contributions on the health of a population.

To address this challenge, the Centre for Public Health within the University of New South Wales, Sydney, Australia, developed an undergraduate course as part of the general education programme targeted to multidisciplinary students in fields other than health. The course objectives are promotion of understanding of the care continuum, comprehension of personal determinants of health as well as global issues affecting health, and appreciation of the potential contribution various professions interacting can have on the health of others in the larger community. This is a step forward in building the capacity of organizations to collaborate intersectorally by educating the future professionals.

CUBA:

Providing population-based care/Working across the care continuum and in primary health care-led systems [99]

In 1984, the Cuban government introduced a family doctor programme with the intention of improving access to health care for the population. Each family doctor is responsible for the general health of the entire population in a small, defined area. These physicians provide preventive, maternal and curative services to children and adults, and monitor patients with chronic

(Continued on next page...)

(Continued from previous page)

conditions. The physicians live in the communities that they serve, often sharing the same apartment block as their patients. Frequently, their consulting room is located in the building in which they live.

In addition to medical consultations, Cuba's family doctors play an active role in promoting health in their communities. They provide informal advice and counselling to community members, and facilitate prevention and self-management groups. They also set a positive example for their patients in the conduct of their day-to-day lives.

Family doctors work closely with nurses in their defined communities. They also collaborate with

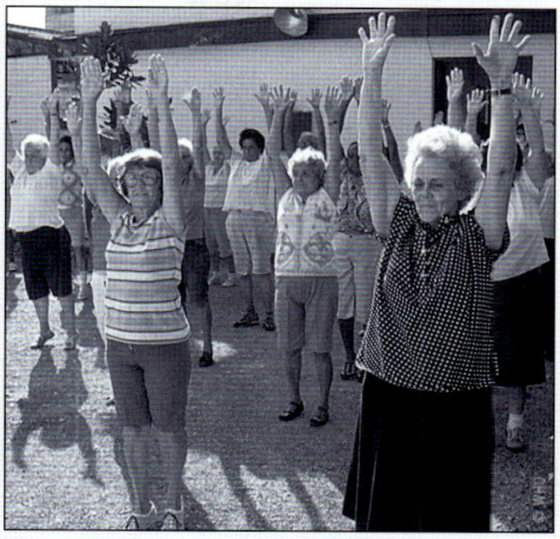

physician specialists, health education workers, and hospital-based social workers in order to coordinate care as it relates to individual patients and their defined population.

New Zealand:

Providing population-based care/Working in primary health care-led systems (100, 101)

The New Zealand Primary Health Care Strategy, launched in 2001, provides a clear direction for primary health care services in the country. The strategy outlines how a new approach to primary health care will improve the health of the population through:

- greater emphasis on population health, health promotion and preventative care
- community involvement
- involving a range of professionals and encouraging multidisciplinary approaches to decision-making
- improving accessibility, affordability and appropriateness of services
- improving coordination and continuity of care
- providing and funding services according to the population's needs (as opposed to fee for services when people are unwell).

The Ministry of Health is working with the health sector to progressively implement the strategy over the next few years.

The Counties Manukau District Health Board also adopted a Chronic Care Management model in 2001. Key components of the model are the targeting of high-risk patients, organization of cost-effective interventions into a system of care, and automated flags and reminders to prompt action. Return on investment analysis suggested potential savings from $277 to $980 per person per annum.

(Case studies continue on next page. . .)

Public health perspective

Spain:

Systems thinking/Working across the care continuum and in primary health care-led systems (102, 103)

In 2000, the Integrated Care Programme for Chronic Patients (ICCP) was conceived as a key component of the restructuring process of one of the tertiary hospitals of the city of Barcelona, Spain *(Hospital Clínic)*. It was developed in response to the challenges posed to the European health care systems by the ageing population and the parallel increase in chronic conditions and health care costs. The situation has been especially dramatic in Spain, where demographic projections indicate that people aged 65 and older will rise from 17% in 2000 to 20% in 2020. Because this scenario has been even more problematic in the Barcelona area, the Catalan Health Administration has supported the ICCP initiative since its initial implementation.

The aim of the project is to develop an open system with a patient-centred model of care. The two driving forces of this ongoing process are: reinforcement of the collaboration among different levels of care through common programmes, and promotion of excellence in biomedical research in the area.

ICCP was planned as a functional unit (Chronic Care Unit) with activities across different clinical institutes of the hospital. One of the unit's pivotal roles is to promote bridging between hospital and primary care services through a continuum of care supported by a web-based information platform.

Core activities of ICCP are:

- validation of innovative health care services based in the home
- support of interactions among health care professionals across the health care system (e.g., primary care, general hospitals, hospices)
- facilitation of accessibility of target patient groups.

Until the end of 2003, ICCP was developed as a set of disease-specific clinical pilots essentially addressed to cover chronic respiratory patients at risk or in early COPD stages to those with end-stage disease. The most prominent programme benefits during the period have been the development of:

- telemedicine/collaborative tools to support the extensive use of spirometry at the primary care level
- innovative home-based services to prevent hospitalization
- home-hospitalization trials
- strategies for end-stage disease.

During 2004, ICCP is being consolidated by expanding the services to other areas of the region, and by adding cardiovascular disorders, diabetes, geriatrics and HIV/AIDS.

Successful outcomes of ICCP have been the empowerment of health care providers at the primary care level, as well as the positive impact on patients' self-management and health-related quality of life.

Conclusions

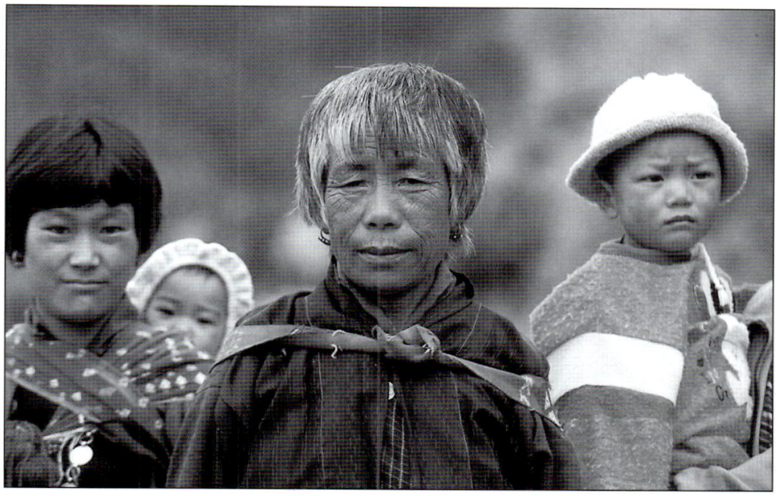

© WORLD BANK

The transition from acute to chronic health problems places a new and different set of demands on the health care workforce. In addition to skills that facilitate the diagnosis and treatment of acute illness and injury, today's workforce needs a core set of competencies that will yield better outcomes for patients with chronic conditions. A workforce for the 21st century must emphasize management over cure, and long-term over episodic care.

This document identifies a core set of competencies to improve care for chronic conditions:

- The essence of this care is to *centre on the patient*. This is a shift from traditional, provider-focused practice, and it requires the workforce to develop communication skills that empower patients through seeing health from the patient's perspective, and motivating and training patients in health-related self-management.
- Solo practice is no longer adequate to achieve positive outcomes for chronic problems; the workforce must be capable of creating and maintaining *partnerships* with everyone involved: patients and their families, other providers and the community.
- The workforce needs skills that ensure continuous *quality improvement* in terms of patient safety and service delivery efficiency.

- The ability to use available *information and communication technology* is essential in caring for patients with problems that persist across time, providers and settings.
- Finally, the workforce needs the ability to view health care from a broad, *public health perspective,* which will enable them to understand their responsibility and accountability within the larger health care system.

The health care workforce is among the most important factors in the health care system. They are instrumental in stimulating, implementing, and maintaining change to improve care for chronic conditions. Consequently, educational reform for this group is essential. Improvements in their preparation and training will require the commitment of a broad-based partnership. Genuine educational reform will not be possible without concerted and sustained efforts among decision-makers, academic leaders and health-related professional bodies.

References

1. *Innovative care for chronic conditions: Building blocks for action*. Geneva, World Health Organization, 2002.
2. Institute of Medicine. *Health professions education: A bridge to quality*. Washington DC, The National Academies Press, 2003.
3. Institute of Medicine. *Improving medical education: Enhancing the behavioral and social science content of medical school curricula*. Washington DC, The National Academies Press, 2004.
4. O'Neil EH and the Pew Health Professions Commission. *Creating health professional practice for a new century*. San Francisco, Pew Health Professions Commission, 1998.
5. *Definition of competency*. Washington DC, Pan American Health Organization, 2002.
6. *World Health Report 2004. Changing history*. Geneva, World Health Organization, 2004.
7. *World Health Report 2002. Reducing risks, promoting healthy life*. Geneva, World Health Organization, 2002.
8. *Human resources and national health systems: Shaping the agenda for action*. Geneva, World Health Organization, 2002.
9. *Making medical practice and education more relevant to peoples' needs: The contribution of the family doctor*. Geneva, World Health Organization, 1994.
10. Griner P. The workforce for health: Response. In: Institute of Medicine. *2020 vision: Health in the 21st century*. Washington DC, National Academies Press, 1996:102–107.
11. Institute of Medicine. *Crossing the quality chasm: A new health system for the 21st century*. Washington DC, National Academies Press, 2001.
12. *Physician concerns: Caring for people with chronic conditions*. Baltimore, Partnership for Solutions, 2002 (http://www.partnershipforsolutions.org/DMS/files/2002/physicianccern.pdf, accessed 22 October 2004).
13. Wagner EH et al. A survey of leading chronic disease management programs: Are they consistent with the literature? *Managed Care Quarterly*, 1999, 7:55–66.
14. Von Korff M, Tiemens B. Individualized stepped care for chronic illness. *Western Journal of Medicine*, 2000, 172:133–137.
15. American College of Rheumatology guidelines. *Arthritis and Rheumatism*, 1996, 39:713–722.
16. Agency for Health Care Policy and Research (AHCPR). *Depression in primary care. Vol. 2 Treatment of major depression*. Rockville, MD, Public Health Service, 1993 (Publication 93–0551).
17. AHCPR. *Heart failure: Evaluation and care of patients with left ventricular systolic dysfunction (Clinical Practice Guideline No. 11)*. Rockville, Public Health Service, 1994.
18. *National Asthma Education Program guidelines*. Bethesda, National Asthma Education Program, Office of Prevention, Education, and Control, National Heart, Lung and Blood Institute, National Institutes of Health, 1991 (Publication 91–3042).

19. American Diabetes Association. American Diabetes Association guidelines. *Diabetes Care*, 1999, 22:S32–S41.

20. Steering Committee and Membership of the Advisory Council to Improve Outcomes Nationwide in Heart Failure. Consensus recommendations for the management of chronic heart failure. *American Journal of Cardiology*, 1999, 83:1A–31A.

21. Bodenheimer T, Wagner EH, Grumbach K. Improving primary care for patients with chronic illness. The Chronic Care Model, Part 2. *Journal of the American Medical Association*, 2002, 288:1909–1914.

22. Von Korff M et al. Collaborative management of chronic illness: Essential elements. *Annals of Internal Medicine*, 1997, 127:1097–1102.

23. McWhinney I. The need for transformed clinical method. In: M. Stewart, D Roter, eds. *Communicating with medical patients*. London, Sage, 1989.

24. *The European definition of general practice/family medicine*. Barcelona, World Organization of Family Doctors (WONCA), 2002.

25. *American College of Graduate Medical Education general competencies*. Chicago, American College of Graduate Medical Education, 1999. (http://www.acgme.org/outcome/comp/compFull.asp, accessed 22 October 2004).

26. *FIP statement of professional standards. Code of ethics for pharmacists*. The Hague, International Pharmaceutical Federation (FIP), 1997.

27. *ICN framework of competencies for the generalist nurse*. Geneva, International Council of Nurses, 2003.

28. *FIP statement of professional standards. Pharmaceutical care*. International Pharmaceutical Federation (FIP), 1998.

29. *Declaration of Lisbon on the rights of the patient*. Ferney-Voltaire, World Medical Association, 1995. (http://www.wma.net/e/policy/l4.htm, accessed 22 October 2004).

30. Delbanco TL, Daley J. Through the patient's eyes: Strategies toward more successful contraception. *Obstetrics and Gynaecology*, 1996, 88:415–425.

31. Lorig K. Self-management of chronic illness: A model for the future. *Generations,* 1993, Fall:11–14.

32. Goldberg RJ, Novack DH. Psychosocial review of systems. *Social Science and Medicine*, 1992, 35:261–269.

33. Kundahl K. Cultural diversity: An evolving challenge to physician-patient communication. *Journal of the American Medical Association*, 2003, 289:94.

34. *Eradicating low health literacy: The first public health movement of the 21st century*. New York, Pfizer Partnership for Clear Health Communication, 2003, (http://www.aameda.org/MemberServices/Exec/Articles/sum03/EradicatingLowHealthcareLiteracy.pdf, accessed 22 October 2004).

35. McGinnis JM, Foege WH. Actual causes of death in the United States. *Journal of the American Medical Association*, 1993, 270:2207–2212.

36. Bodenheimer T, Lorig K, Holman H. Patient self-management of chronic disease in primary care. *Journal of the American Medical Association*, 2002, 288:2469–2475.

37. Beresford SA et al. A dietary intervention in primary care practice: The eating pattern study. *American Journal of Public Health*, 1997, 87:6610–6616.

38. Nawaz H, Adams ML, Katz DL. Physician-patient interactions regarding diet, exercise and smoking. *Preventive Medicine*, 2000, 31:652–657.

39. Miller WR, Rollnick S, eds. *Motivational interviewing: Preparing people to change addictive behaviour, 2nd ed*. New York, Guilford, 2002.

40. Mead N, Bower P. Patient centeredness: A conceptual framework and review of the empirical literature. *Social Science and Medicine*, 2000, 51:1087–1110.

41. Bourbeau J et al. Reduction of hospital utilization in patients with chronic obstructive pulmonary disease: a disease-specific self-management intervention. *Archives of Internal Medicine,* 2003, 163:585–590.

42. Fu D et al. Implementation and quantitative evaluation of chronic disease self-management programme in Shanghai, China: randomized controlled trial. *Bulletin of the World Health Organization*, 2003, 81:174--82.

43. Sorenson WB et al. A visit to a Mexican specialty hospital: The patient as leader? *Hospital Topics: Research and Perspectives on Health Care*, Vol. 78, no. 1 Winter 2000, 10–13.

44. *The Integrated Management of Adolescent and Adult Illness modules.* Geneva, World Health Organization, 2004. (http://www.who.int/3by5/publications/documents/imai/en/, accessed 22 October 2004).

45. *The working partnership (Book 1). The value of partnerships*. London, National Health Service, Health Development Agency, 2000.

46. Essential elements of communication in medical encounters: The Kalamazoo consensus statement (Bayer-Fetzer Conference on Physician-Patient Communication in Medical Education). *Academic Medicine*, 2001, 76:390–393.

47. Szasz T, Hollender M. A contribution to the philosophy of medicine: The basic models of the doctor-patient relationship. *Archives of Internal Medicine*, 1956, 97:585–592.

48. Kaplan S, Greenfield S, Ware J. Assessing the effects of physician-patient interactions on the outcomes of chronic disease. *Medical Care,* 1989, 27: s110–s127.

49. Grol R et al. Disease-centred versus patient-centred attitudes: Comparison of general practitioners in Belgium, Britain, and The Netherlands. *Family Practice*, 1990, 7:100–103.

50. Halpern R et al. A synthesis of nine major reports on physicians' competencies for the emerging practice environment. *Academic Medicine*, 2001, 76:606–615.

51. Bush J. Recommendations for the future of family medicine. *Family Practice Management*, 2004, 11:34–38.

52. Wagner EH. The role of patient care teams in chronic disease management. *British Medical Journal*, 2000, 320:569–572.

53. Wagner EH, Austin,BT, Von Korff M. Organizing care for patients with chronic illness. *Milbank Quarterly*, 1996, 74:511–544.

54. Wagner EH. Chronic disease management: What will it take to improve care for chronic illness? *Effective Clinical Practice*, 1998, 1:2–4.

55. Calkins E et al., eds. *New ways to care for older people*. New York, Springer, 1998.

56. Holman H, Lorig K. Patients as partners in managing chronic disease. Partnership as a prerequisite for effective and efficient health care. *British Medical Journal*, 2000, 320, 525–527.

57. Glasgow RE , Wagner EH, Kaplan S et al. If diabetes is a public health problem, why not treat it as one? A population based approach to chronic illness. *Annals of Behavioural Medicine*, 1999, 21:159–170.

58. Future of Family Medicine Project Leadership Committee. The future of family medicine: A collaborative project of the family medicine community. *Annals of Family Medicine*, 2004, 2:S3–S32.

59. Hoy WE et al, Reducing premature death and renal failure in Australian Aborigines: A community-based cardiovascular and renal programme. *Medical Journal of Australia,* 172:473–478, 2000.

60. *The Diabetes Programme for Pharmacies.* Tampere, The Association of Finnish Pharmacies and the Finnish Diabetes Association, 2001.

61. *Report of the First International Review Meeting. Practical Approach to Lung Health strategy, Rabat, 4–6 September 2002*. World Health Organization, 2003 (WHO/CDS /TB/2003.324). (http://whqlibdoc.who.int/hq/2003/WHO_CDS_TB_2003.324.pdf, accessed 22 October 2004).

62. *Collaborative practice in the 21st century.*, Geneva, International Council of Nurses, 2004.

63. *Declaration with guidelines for continuous quality improvement in health care*. Ferney-Voltaire, World Medical Association, 1997.

64. Berwick DM. A primer on leading the improvement of systems. *British Medical Journal*, 1996, 312:619–622.

65. Holman WL et al. Alabama coronary artery bypass grafting project: Results of a state-wide quality improvement initiative. *Journal of the American Medical Association*, 2001, 285:3003–3010.

66. Kiefe CI et al. Improving quality improvement using achievable benchmarks for physician feedback: A randomized controlled trial. *Journal of the American Medical Association*, 2001, 285:2871–2879.

67. O'Connor GT et al. A regional intervention to improve the hospital mortality associated with coronary artery bypass graft surgery. The Northern New England Cardiovascular Disease Study Group. *Journal of the American Medical Association*, 1996, 275:841–846.

68. Berwick DM, Enthoven A, Bunker JP. Quality management in the NHS: The doctor's role – II. *British Medical Journal*, 1992, 304:304–308.

69. Mutha S, Norman G, O'Neil E. Medical Practice 2002: How we get there. *Western Journal of Medicine*, 2000, 172:274–277.

70. *Veracruz Initiative for diabetes awareness (VIDA Project).* Washington DC, Pan American Health Organization, 2004. (http://www.paho.org/english/ad/dpc/nc/dia-vida-veracruz.htm, accessed 19 October 2004).

71. *Report of the consultative meeting on primary health care policy review in the Eastern Mediterranean Region, Muscat, Oman, 28–30 January 2002*. Muscat, Sultanate of Oman Ministry of Health, 2002.

72. *Annual Health Report 2000 A.D. 1420–1421 A.H.* Muscat, Directorate General of Planning, Sultanate of Oman Ministry of Health, 2001.

73. *Global strategy for the diagnosis, management, and prevention of chronic obstructive pulmonary disease: NHLBI/WHO Workshop.* Ghent, Global Initiative for Chronic Obstructive Lung Disease, 2001.

74. Enright PL, Kaminsky DA. Strategies for screening for chronic obstructive pulmonary disease. *Respiratory Care,* 2003, 48:1194–1201.

75. Berwick DM. Lessons from developing nations on improving health care. *British Medical Journal,* 2004, 328:1124–1129.

76. Forsstrom J, Rigby M. TEAC-Health: Research-based recommendations for European certification of health telematics services. *Studies in Health Technology and Informatics*, 2000, 77:288–292.

77. *World Health Report 2001. Mental health: New understanding new hope.* Geneva, World Health Organization, 2001.

78. *Africa telecom projections, 1995–2005.* International Telecommunication Union, April, 2004. (http://www.itu.int/ITU-D/afr/statistics/projections.htm, accessed 27 October 2004).

79. Cornish PA et al. Rural interdisciplinary mental health team building via satellite: a demonstration project. *Telemedicine Journal and e-health: the official journal of the American Telemedicine Association*. 2003, 9:63–71.

80. Mudur G. The great technological divide. *British Medical Journal,* 2004, 328:788.

81. *Uganda Health Information Network*. Watertown, Satellife, 2004. (http://pda.healthnet.org/index.php, accessed 22 October 2004).

82. Young M et al. A Telephone-linked computer system for COPD care. *Chest*, 2001, 119:1565–1575.

83. *Public health management*. Geneva, World Health Organization, 2002.

84. Acheson D. *Public health in England. The report of the committee of inquiry into the future development of the public health function*. London, HMSO, 1988.

85. Rivo ML. It's time to start practicing population-based health care. *Family Practice Management*, 1998, 5:37–46.

86. Boland P, ed. *Redesigning health care delivery*. Boland Health Care, Berkeley, 1996, 159–163.

87. Zeich R. Patient identification as a key to population health management. *New Medicine*, 1998, 2:109–116.

88. Beck A et al. A randomized trial of group outpatient visits for chronically ill older HMO members: The Cooperative Health Care Clinic. *Journal of the American Geriatrics Society*, 1997, 45:543–549.

89. Wasson J et al. Telephone care as a substitute for routine clinic follow-up. *Journal of the American Medical Association*, 1992, 267:1828–1829.

90. Maisiak R, Austin J, Heck L. Health outcomes of two telephone interventions for patients with rheumatoid arthritis or osteoarthritis. *Arthritis and Rheumatism*, 1996, 19:1391–1399.

91. el Ansari W et al. New skills for a new age: leading the introduction of public health concepts in healthcare curricula. *Public Health*, 2003,117:77–87.

92. *National Public Health Leadership Institute (PHLI) programme model, 2004*. Chapel Hill, National Public Health Leadership Institute, 2004. (http://www.phli.org/aboutPHLI/index.htm, accessed 19 October 2004).

93. Aronson D, *Overview of systems thinking. 1996–8*. (http://www.thinking.net/Systems_Thinking/OverviewSTarticle.pdf, accessed 19 October 2004).

94. Plsek PE, Greenhalgh T. The challenge of complexity in health care. *British Medical Journal*, 2001, 323:625–628.

95. *From Alma-Ata to the year 2000: Reflections at the midpoint*. Geneva, World Health Organization, 1988.

96. *World Health Report 2003. Shaping the future*. Geneva, World Health Organization, 2003.

97. Declaration of Alma-Ata. In: *International Conference on Primary Health Care, Alma-Ata, USSR, 6–12 September 1978*. Geneva, World Health Organization, 1978.

98. Furber WE, Ritchie JE. Spreading the word: Teaching health promotion to students from disciplines other than health. *Education for Health*, 2000, 13:329–336.

99. Warman A. Living the revolution: Cuban health workers. *Journal of Clinical Nursing*, 2001, 10:311–319.

100. *Primary health care strategy*. Wellington, New Zealand Ministry of Health, 2001. (http://www.moh.govt.nz/primaryhealthcare, accessed 22 October 2004).

101. Wellingham J et al. The development and implementation of the Chronic Care Management Programme in Counties Manukau. *New Zealand Medical Journal*, 2003, 116:U327.

102. Hernandez C et al. CHRONIC project: Home hospitalisation of exacerbated chronic obstructive pulmonary disease patients. *European Respiratory Journal*. 2003, 21:58–67.

103. Roca J et al. Home management of exacerbations of chronic obstructive pulmonary disease. In: NM Siafakas, NR Anthonisen, D Georgopoulos, eds. *Acute exacerbation of chronic obstructive pulmonary disease (part VII chapter 1)*. In the series Lung Biology in Health and Disease (Claude Lenfant, ed), New York, Marcel Dekker Inc, 2002.